THE HEART REVOLUTION

Dr Paul Sherwood, consultant in physical medicine, trained at Cambridge University and the Westminster Hospital. After achieving a degree in medicine he worked as a house surgeon at Westminster Hospital, and later at Barts before becoming a consultant at a number of hospitals.

Dr Sherwood set up his own private clinic in London where he has been developing his own form of physical medicine over a period of 40 years.

Also by Dr Paul Sherwood
THE BACK AND BEYOND

THE HEART REVOLUTION

Dr Paul Sherwood

ARROW

Published by Arrow Books in 1994

1 3 5 7 9 10 8 6 4 2

Copyright © Dr Paul Sherwood 1994
Illustrations by Ian Cumming

The right of Paul Sherwood has been asserted under the
Copyright, Designs and Patents Act, 1988 to be identified as
the author of this work

Arrow Books Limited
Random House, 20 Vauxhall Bridge Road
London, SW1V 2SA

Random House Australia (Pty) Limited
20 Alfred Street, Milsons Point, Sydney
New South Wales 2061, Australia

Random House New Zealand Limited
18 Poland Road, Glenfield
Auckland 10, New Zealand

Random House South Africa (Pty) Limited
PO Box 337, Bergvlei, South Africa

Random House UK Limited Reg. No. 954009

A CIP catalogue record for this book is available
from the British Library

ISBN 0 09 943151 3

Phototypeset by Intype, London
Printed and bound in Great Britain by
Cox & Wyman Ltd, Reading, Berks.

DEDICATION

To my grandchild Emily who so warmed the cockles of my heart that it made me feel young enough to write this book.

CONTENTS

ACKNOWLEDGEMENTS

To Mary Atkinson who has taken my disorderly thoughts and regimented them into a readable form – for her enthusiasm and understanding of my ideas and her encouragement to convert them into a book. To my family who have suffered greatly through the birth pangs without complaining, and to my staff and friends who have helped in the book's preparation, have read the manuscript and have produced many of the ideas incorporated in this volume.

ACKNOWLEDGEMENTS

FOREWORD

The Back and Beyond dealt with problems with the back and also other diseases that are caused by back trouble. It did, however, deliberately have a major omission – the influence of bad backs on coronary thrombosis. This was because I thought that the subject might become clouded in the mass of information contained in the book. It seemed important to me that the link between back trouble and heart disease should be dealt with separately so it could be seen as a story of hope and not a chronicle of alarm and despair. It was also important, I thought, to have enough elbow room to explain the theme of coronary problems sufficiently clearly that it would not cause panic in every person suffering a few twinges in their back.

We all know that eating too much (and eating the wrong food), smoking and taking too little exercise diminishes our expectation of life – yet many people continue to do so without worrying at all. Why then should people be frightened by news of another potential cause of increased risk, especially as this cause is capable of being reasonably easily rectified? This book shows how dealing with the problem can greatly reduce the risk to the heart and, at the same time, diminish the effects of other known harmful factors.

AUTHOR'S NOTE

This book explains a new concept in the cause and treatment of coronary thrombosis. The subject matter applies only to those people who have recovered from heart attacks or have never had one. It is in no way intended to replace or modify the orthodox medical treatment of a heart attack itself.

INTRODUCTION

'NEWS FLASH – there has been another major train disaster in Britain, killing 486 people and seriously injuring around 800. This is the 365th such crash in the last 12 months – there's been one every single day this year.'

Can you imagine the public outcry and the stupendous amount of resources that would be put into rectifying this horrifying situation? Yet this is the scale of devastation caused by coronary heart disease in Britain alone and which continues despite the efforts of the world's medical practitioners. It is because of this that I feel justified in putting forward the ideas in this book in the hope that it may help diminish these appalling figures. Here are two more: in Britain, 35,000,000 working days are lost each year, at an annual cost to the Health Service of £70,000,000.

Without doubt, heart research has achieved many successes. The knowledge of the medical profession concerning both prevention and treatment is one of the miracles of modern times. However, heart disease is still Britain's biggest killer and disabler, and researchers are still looking for clues to many outstanding anomalies.

To most people, coronary thrombosis seems a straightforward affair – an artery supplying the heart muscle becomes blocked by a clot, the heart suffers shock and may go into major dysfunction and, in the end, the heart and the victim will recover or not, according to the circumstances. But on closer inspection it is not as simple a story as this.

Pause for a moment ... Remember when that famous person was reported to have died suddenly of a heart attack? Wasn't there some mention of a visit to the doctor some hours or even a day before because he was feeling unwell? Maybe he had even been advised to stop work and take it easy for a day. Did he *know* he was nearing a sudden clotting of his coronary artery?

- Why, when the severity of their arterial disease remains at a constant level, does someone have a heart attack at three o'clock in the morning, then another several months later? How can you account for these periods between attacks when the level of disease in the arterial wall remains unchanged?
- Why are other arteries in the body – just as diseased as the coronary artery – hardly ever subject to a thrombosis?
- Why is it that, occasionally, when people who have suffered a massive heart attack arrive at hospital; the tests they are given, even the electrocardiogram (ECG), can be completely normal? This would not have been the case if a permanent clot was the cause.
- Why, in some instances, does a myocardial infarct – the death of part of the heart muscle because the blood supply to it has been cut off; commonly called a 'heart attack' – precede a coronary thrombosis? Sometimes the clot in the coronary artery is found at post-mortem to have formed *after* the death of the patient. This means that it could not have been the clot that caused the fatal attack.

2

- Why do patients show signs such as tiredness, transient dizziness and indigestion for several years before a coronary thrombosis – and yet all tests are normal?

A simple thrombosis (clot) in a coronary artery does not explain any of these phenomena. A spasm of the artery (a violent contraction of the ring of muscles in the artery wall) can explain some of them, but not, for instance, why the patient feels ill long before the attack. But a consideration of why the artery should go into a spasm and then possibly clot will lead you back to a consideration of the nerves transmitting impulses to these arteries and, finally, to a consideration of a controlling 'nerve computer' called the *stellate ganglion*. This can provide the answers to these anomalies.

The Heart Revolution answers all these questions with one single and logical explanation. The starting point of the coronary problem is an old injury which disturbed the spinal column and damaged its facet joints. Although there may be no apparent symptoms for many years, the repercussions throughout the whole body are serious. The jolt caused by the injury sends the muscles across the facet joints into a protective spasm. The spasm increases the supply of blood to the muscles but reduces the efficiency of the muscle pump. As a result of poor pumping action, congestion builds up in the tissue spaces. The congestion spreads and upsets effective circulation in the adjacent tissues. Some of the most important of these comprise the sympathetic nerve chain which lies close to the spinal muscles in the lower neck and upper thoracic part of the spine.

The sympathetic nerve chain works in opposition to the parasympathetic nerve chain, each balancing the other. If the sympathetic is not functioning correctly, this equilibrium is upset. Low sympathetic drive can have far-reaching effects on the normal functioning of the body systems – including, and most importantly in the context of this book, the coronary arteries which provide the heart muscle with an essential supply of blood.

I will be describing the stellate ganglion – a controlling part of the sympathetic nerve system – and its functions, following this with a detailed analysis of the cause of its malfunction, which can lead to a coronary spasm. I will show why the stellate ganglion commonly causes problems ranging from headaches, Reynaud's disease, tiredness and low blood pressure, and yet its effect on the coronary arteries is comparatively rare.

This theory, which concentrates on the involvement of the sympathetic nerve chain with back injuries, offers exciting possibilities in the field of coronary prevention, including an early warning system – making it possible to pinpoint the signs of vulnerability to a heart attack in the preceding weeks, months and even years. These symptoms, such as tiredness, neck trouble, indigestion, dizzy attacks and anxiety, would not normally be associated with an imminent heart attack.

Knowing that a risk may be present makes it possible to offer reasonably effective, yet simple treatment for the prevention of the attack, which involves physical medicine that can be given by any therapist including those working within the National Health Service. Furthermore, those people who have already had a coronary episode can benefit from the same treatment, which lessens the probability of another attack. As well as offering protection to the heart, patients will also notice a dramatic improvement in their general health.

This book has been written as a message of hope, that it will add an extra dimension to the prevention of coronary attacks. I would like to stress that my recommended treatment is not an alternative to conventional, orthodox medicine. The specialized care following a coronary episode is outside the scope of this book, as I believe that there is no substitute for the expert advice and treatment given by cardiologists. What this book provides is a unique theory based on medical principles which offers both a diagnosis and treatment for coronary disease.

The contents of the book are based on a paper which was originally written in 1958. However, despite the fact that heart attacks account for one third of all the deaths in this country, publication in medical journals was totally blocked. My first book, *The Back and Beyond*, has been criticized by some medical quarters that the subject should properly have been published in the form of scientific papers in recognized medical journals, but if editors refuse to publish papers, how can there be any debate on their validity? Now my theories have been published in book form, they are available for open discussion.

1
THE MIRACLE PUMP

The heart is an amazingly sophisticated piece of equipment for supplying the body with energy. Indeed, its mechanics are so clever that they are easy to take for granted. To show just how often the power and efficiency of the heart are overlooked, I would like to repeat a conversation with one of my patients.

Some years ago, a junior minister of power mentioned to me that he was studying alternative methods of obtaining energy for when oil and coal ran out. He described several very elaborate and costly methods of using the Earth's resources for power, including drilling a hole three miles deep in Cornwall, pouring water on to the red hot rocks at the bottom and getting back enough steam for a generator to produce sufficient electricity to light a few houses.

Rather tongue in cheek, I replied that this didn't seem a very economical way of solving the problems of the future. Wouldn't it be a more profitable line of research to look into a pump that I knew about? This pump works on a dilute sugar solution for its energy and is capable of filling an average-sized bath in about four minutes. What's more, the pump itself *and* enough fuel for about three weeks could be contained in a tin considerably smaller than a one-gallon petrol can. The minister was rather taken aback and said that he was sure no such pump existed because, if it did, he would know all about it. Then I told him *which* pump I was talking about – the heart.

The Cardiovascular System

The heart is at the centre of the body's circulation. Before discussing its role and functions I would like to step back in time to when life started on Earth and thus address the very fundamental question of why we need a cardiovascular system at all.

Life began in the sea with single amoeba-like cells (*see* Fig. 1.1). These absorbed oxygen and food from the water and excreted waste products into the sea. Gradually, as these cells became more sophisticated, they joined together (*see* Fig. 1.2) and were able to ingest larger particles and

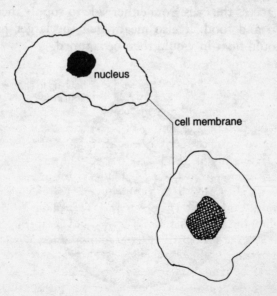

Figure 1.1   Single cells – amoeba

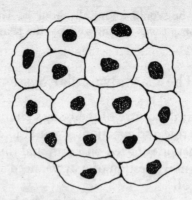

Figure 1.2 Cells forming a plate

even single cells. Over the millennia, the flat plates of cells developed into spheres (*see* Fig. 1.3), each with an opening that allowed sea water to enter. This meant that the sea could access the cells from either side to supply them with oxygen and food. It also meant that the larger particles that could float in would then be trapped.

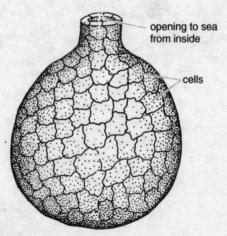

Figure 1.3 Cells forming a sphere with an opening

8

After some while the 'hole' in the sphere turned into a tube which took in food at one end and pushed out waste at the other. This enabled specialized 'digestive and collection' devices to be contrived and the cell colony's efficiency in collecting food was increased considerably. Nerve networks developed between the cells which enabled co-ordination of movement but all this time, each cell relied directly on the sea for its supply of oxygen and food.

The interdependence of the cells became greater and greater, with a central brain developing which further increased the efficiency of the organism by providing an overall control of strategy. The limit of development and complexity was probably reached with the flatworm, which had to remain flat because it was so important for each cell to be close to the sea water. Very small roundworms could also develop, but anything bigger would result in cells living too far from the water in the sea to be able to get adequate supplies from it.

DEVELOPMENT OF THE HEART

Then suddenly liberation was achieved. The worm developed a system of pipes which branched all over its body so that no cell was more than a minute distance from this system. Insects still use this mechanism to transmit air all over their bodies. Then a heart developed that pumped sea water around the worm.

It is likely that the primitive tubes gradually turned into a closed circulatory system that held sea water to bathe all the cells in the organism. This had several advantages: the pipes could take the fluid far greater distances; no foreign bodies could waft into the tubes and block them; and the pipes could no longer act as a pathway to hostile organisms entering the system. Also, as the tubes no longer needed to be large for diffusion, they could now be graded in size, according to need, from a main trunk to tiny twigs.

THE SEA IN OUR BLOOD

The salty fluid that bathes our own cells and, indeed, that circulates throughout our bodies is exactly the same composition as the sea – with, of course, the addition of the three special factors: the oxygen-carrying *red cells*; the soldier-scavenger *white cells* which engulf foreign bodies, bacteria and viruses; and the *platelets* which help to stop bleeding and are the trigger of the body's clotting mechanism. So when we climbed out of the sea on to dry land, we did, in fact, take the sea with us.

Over the years, the sea has become more concentrated due to the rivers flowing into it taking in salt from the land, and at the same time because of the evaporation of the water from the sea by the heat of the sun, so our blood is not as dense as sea water is today. It is interesting to note that scientists, knowing the time it takes for a given increase in the concentration in the sea, use this difference in the sea's salt level to date when sea creatures actually came on to dry land some 350 million years ago.

The Heart of the Matter

The heart has developed considerably from those early days. In its latest development in human beings, it is a double pump or, to be more precise, two pumps within one single unit (*see* Fig. 1.4 and Fig 1.6). The two sides of the heart are separated from each other but pump in unison. The highly accurate synchronization of the two pumps is vital to the efficient working of the system.

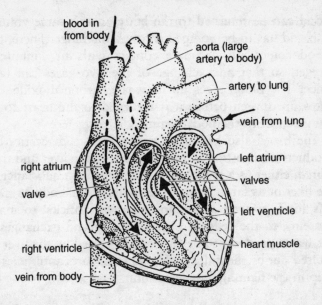

Figure 1.4 Heart to show chambers and vessels

The heart pumps oxygen-rich blood throughout the body to carry this essential gas to all the tissues. This output of blood is largely controlled by the amount of blood that flows back into the heart from your body and varies considerably according to how much exercise you are taking. The higher the level of activity, the faster the blood circulates in your body. When you are running in a race your body may need as much as 25 litres (5½ gal.) of blood a minute; when you are asleep 4 litres (1 gal.) is adequate. The actual quantity of blood circulating varies as well, but this is controlled by other mechanisms in the body.

When the blood returns to the heart, it lacks oxygen and is loaded with carbon dioxide, which is the product of cell combustion. This must be corrected before the blood can be returned to the body, so this same volume of blood has to be pumped through the lungs. There, the blood comes into intimate contact with air containing oxygen so that an exchange of the two gases can take place. The blood gives up its waste carbon dioxide and takes up oxygen before it is returned to the heart to be pumped out to the body again.

The blood also has other transport uses. It carries the products of digestion to be processed in the liver and then stored, either as a readily available sugar-like substance in the liver or as fat in many other parts of the body. It takes this food, as well as amino acids (the 'bricks' to make protein), to the cells all over the body and exchanges it for waste products to be either reprocessed by the liver or filtered out by the kidneys. It also transports antibodies to help in the fight against infection.

A FAIR EXCHANGE

To ensure an adequate transfer of oxygen and carbon dioxide between the air and the blood, the lungs are cleverly arranged to create a large exchange area. The smallest air passages terminate in little thin-walled balloons or pockets called alveoli (*alveus*=a cavity, *alveolus*=a small cavity). The walls of each alveolus contain a massive network of blood vessels so that the blood comes as close as possible to the air (*see* Fig. 1.5). If all these little pockets were spread out flat, they would cover the area of a full-sized tennis court with all its surrounds. It's incredible how small the lungs are when you consider this.

It is in order to ensure that exactly the same amount of blood goes through both the lungs and the body that the heart is divided into two sides which work in unison, beating at the same speed and pumping out the same

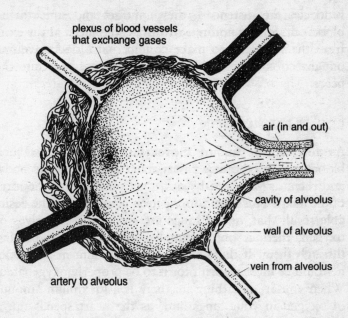

plexus of blood vessels
that exchange gases

air (in and out)

cavity of alveolus

wall of alveolus

vein from alveolus

artery to alveolus

Figure 1.5   Alveolus (unit cavity of the lung)

volume of blood. As Fig. 1.4 shows, each pump has two
hollow chambers: the weak-walled atrium (plural='atria'
– Latin=cavity or entrance hall of a house; also called
'auricle') and the larger, more powerful ventricle (*venter*=
'belly' and *cule* or *icle*='diminished' – i.e. 'small belly').
Blood arrives in the atria which act as collecting reservoirs
and provide temporary accommodation for the constant,
steady stream of blood from the body and the lungs. This
is necessary because the heart, with its intermittent action,
can only take in blood when relaxing after a pumping
contraction.

When one of these contractions occurs, the atria diminish in size squeezing out the blood through non-return
valves into the larger ventricles. In turn, when the larger

13

ventricles are distended, they contract and squeeze the blood out. Strong non-return valves are placed at the exits from the ventricles to make certain that blood travels in one direction only and does not regurgitate back into the heart.

BREATHING ACTION

As you breathe in, the movements of your chest suck blood into the thoracic cavity from the rest of the body, and then, as you breathe out, they push it into the atria of the heart. This respiratory action brings about the desirable result that, as the lungs are emptying themselves of oxygen, there is only a small supply of blood passing through them. If there were a large amount at this time, it would be more difficult for it to be properly oxygenated. When you are breathing in, there is a maximum amount of oxygen in your lungs and, as the heart speeds up, a larger amount of blood to be serviced.

FUNCTIONS OF THE HEART

In fulfilling its role of supplying blood to the lungs and body, the heart carries out two major functions:

- precise control of the quantity of circulating blood
- helping, to a large extent, to maintain an adequate blood pressure for the circumstances.

CONTROL OF BLOOD IN CIRCULATION

All engines need fuel – and your body is no exception. It relies on blood, carrying sugar (the cells' food) and oxygen, from your heart to keep working. However, it is very different to an ordinary engine in that, for all its tremendous power and capabilities, it can survive on a comparatively small amount of fuel.

In other words, the body contains a huge amount of machinery in a very small package. There are the muscles and bones necessary for movement and power; the heart, the vast complex of blood vessels and the associated lungs to act as the gas exchange and transport facility; the brain and the huge nerve networks to guide and operate all systems. Furthermore, in the stomach and intestines the body has the most sophisticated collecting, breaking down and absorption mechanism, an extraordinary chemical processing plant and storage facility in the liver, not to forget the purifying, recycling and secretion abilities of the kidneys and large bowel – and still has room to house sufficient fuel to run this truly astonishing piece of machinery for up to three weeks. Indeed it has been calculated that if humans were to try and design a human body, it would need at least 45.5 litres (80 pints) of circulating blood to carry out the functions that our bodies are capable of achieving with only about 4.5 litres (8 pints). This is thanks to the incredibly sophisticated control of the blood distribution to the capillaries, the minute blood vessels that link arteries and veins, and which carry blood to and from the tissues.

The amount of circulating blood required at any one time varies enormously, depending on the degree of effort the body is making. When you are sleeping, for example, your body's needs are met by only about 4.5 litres (8 pints) of blood circulating every minute, but as soon as you start walking around, more is required. When you run or dance, an even greater amount, even as much as 40 litres (70 pints) of blood must circulate a minute. Pumping at this rate, your heart would be able to fill, from the output of one side alone, an average-sized bath in about four minutes.

ARTERY POWER

Nature has devised a sophisticated mechanism similar to irrigation which enables your heart to alter the supply of blood rapidly and highly accurately, from a small maintenance output to a very big volume which can be sustained over a long period. Thus your body is supplied with exactly the right quantity of blood at exactly the right time. Central to this mechanism are the arteries. As Fig. 1.6 shows, blood leaves the heart through the large artery called the aorta. This artery branches off into smaller arteries which lead to minute arterioles and then to a network of tiny capillaries, thus supplying every part of your body with oxygen and essential nutrients.

The arteries which carry the oxygenated blood to the body have circular muscles in their walls which can vary the internal diameter of the artery. When the muscles contract, the diameter diminishes, and in smaller vessels, the hole may be closed off completely. It is this property that enables a large area of the body to be supplied by a relatively small amount of circulating blood. An area in need is immediately supplied, but the supply is then cut off once the area has had sufficient for both its present and immediate future needs.

HEARTBEAT

When a greater volume of blood is used by the body, the heart pumps faster and deeper to increase the supply. If you have a healthy heart, it will beat around 60 to 70 times a minute when you are resting. The number of beats may rise

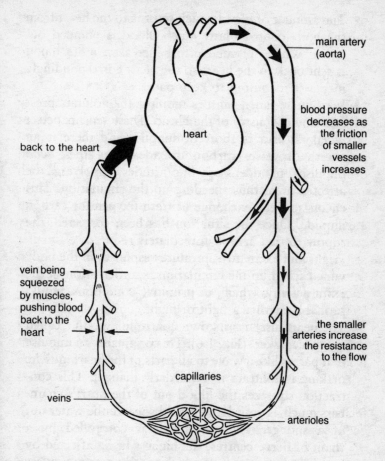

Figure 1.6 The circulation of blood. As blood pressure decreases, the muscles must work to return blood to the heart

to around 160 to 180 a minute when you are taking exercise, and at the same time, the volume of blood pumped at each beat also increases considerably. The heart attains this flexibility by a number of factors, which work together to control both the speed and volume of the beats:

17

- The amount of blood which returns to the heart from the body controls how much blood is pumped out again. When muscular effort increases, more blood is sent back to the heart so the heart correspondingly increases its output to keep pace.
- Very finely tuned sensors monitor the volume, pressure and chemistry of the blood. These sensors detect when an area is short of supplies and there is an excess of waste carbon dioxide. They then send impulses to open up the arteries supplying the affected area, thus speeding up the circulation. This encourages the exchange of fresh oxygen for carbon dioxide. Once the situation has been corrected, the supply to that area is immediately reduced.
- Fright and excitement produce responses in the body which speed up the circulation in anticipation of the extra activity, which, in primitive conditions, would probably involve a fight or flight.
- The heart also has its own controlling nodule called the 'pacemaker' (Fig. 1.6). This originates an impulse that passes like a wave to all parts of the heart muscle, making it contract in an orderly manner. This contraction squeezes the blood out of the heart's chambers much as your hand would squeeze the water out of a sponge. The pacemaker is controlled by a chain of nerve centres, the highest being affected by both emotion and fear, which speed up the impulses produced, and also physical states such as after a meal, when everything slows down.

This control then passes through more primitive centres until it finally affects the pacemaker.

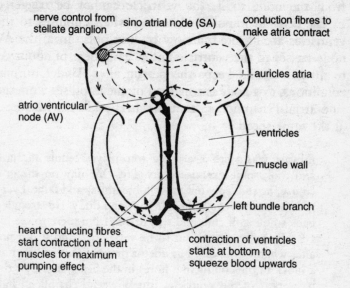

Figure 1.6a The heart. Transmitting fibres and bundles

FAIL-SAFE MECHANISM

We cannot exist without the heart, so the pacemaker maintains the heartbeat when control after control fails. The pacemaker is set at about 100 beats a minute but normally produces only about 60 because it is modified by the nerves controlling it. The impulses from it start the atria contracting and then reach the atrio-ventricular (AV) node. After a sufficient delay to allow the atrial contraction to fill the ventricles, this then triggers off the contraction of the ventricles and ensures that the two beat in effective sequence together (*see* Fig. 1.6).

There is no other contact between the atrium and the ventricle, so in the event of the impulse not passing through the node or down the special conducting material from the node to it, the ventricle cannot be triggered by the original impulse. However, when impulses to the ventricles are blocked, a slow built-in pulse from the AV node passes to the ventricle and a basic beat of about 25 to 40 per second keeps the person alive. Under normal conditions, this node is triggered by the impulses from the sino-atrial (SA) node so that the atria and ventricles beat at the same speed.

Edward was a fit 53-year-old who played tennis and golf and took some exercise every day. One day on the golf course, he suddenly felt unwell, breathless and faint. Every time he tried to walk, he felt faint and dizzy. He struggled back to the golf club and was driven from there to see his GP. His pulse was found to be very slow, and it did not alter whatever he did. His doctor thought that he had had a block in the conducting fibres in the heart, and that the basic beat of the ventricles (the powerful chambers) had taken control as the normal impulses to the atria could now no longer reach them.

An ECG (Electro Cardio Gram) was performed. This test charts the actual electrical impulses generated in the working heart muscle, and by comparing these to those of the normal heart, many abnormal conditions can be accurately diagnosed. Edward's ECG showed that his atria were beating normally but that his ventricles had an independent slow and steady beat.

As a result of this diagnosis, Edward had an electronic pacemaker inserted. This gadget stimulates the ventricles to beat at a normal pace so that the output of the heart is enough for the person to have a nearly normal existence. The newer pacemakers have very long-lasting batteries and are able to vary the speed of the beat to some extent to allow for differing conditions, from rest to exercise. Edward was restored to a virtually normal life.

MAINTAINING CORRECT BLOOD PRESSURE

The heart has a very finely tuned system for ensuring that blood pressure is kept at an adequate level for virtually any situation. It is particularly important that the blood pressure remains relatively constant in the brain. When you are lying down, your brain is at the same height as your heart. When you stand up, your heart suddenly becomes a foot higher so you might expect a drop in blood pressure in the brain and consequent dizziness and fainting. However, the heart corrects the situation almost instantaneously by raising the blood pressure to maintain a constant level in the brain itself. This does not always work sufficiently rapidly.

Ann, aged 24, was typical of many people that I have seen. She had had a nasty fall from a horse when she was 16 years old and, after a few years, began to have numerous aches between her shoulders. She also felt tired much more than seemed normal, but she was particularly worried about the momentary dizzy attacks that she frequently suffered when she stood up from the lying position.

On examination she was found to have, among other things, a somewhat low blood pressure (caused by the bad back) and, also because of her back trouble, her heart was too slow in correcting the fall in pressure to the brain on a change of posture. This caused her to feel dizzy for that moment until the brain pressure was returned to normal. Treatment to her back completely stopped this.

Let us look at how the control of the pressure is achieved. As we have already seen, each time your heart beats – and that's some 100,000 times every day – its muscles contract and blood is pumped out. This blood passes directly into the arterial blood vessels. The walls of the arteries are elastic so they expand to take up this sudden large increase of blood into the system. Between beats, the elasticity of the arteries contracts their walls and this squeezes the blood out of them into the tissues at a uniform speed. If you press gently on the artery in your wrist at the base of your thumb, you can actually feel it expand and relax. This is, of course, your pulse and doctors can tell a great deal about your circulation, blood pressure and heart by feeling and measuring it.

The circular bands of elastic in the arteries all over the body exert a basic pressure on the blood called the diastolic pressure (from the Greek *diastellein*, 'to enlarge or fill') – that is, the pressure in the system while the heart is filling. The high pressure that occurs when a volume of fluid is suddenly forced into the arterial system as the heart contracts is called the systolic pressure (from the Greek *systole*, 'contraction'). This is why your blood pressure is always given in two figures: the top one (say, 120) represents the force of the heart (the systolic pressure), and the lower one (say, 80) is the basic (diastolic) pressure.

The blood leaves the heart through the aorta, the main artery, and then goes into smaller arteries, which branch off and become even smaller (*see* Fig. 1.6). As their size decreases, the resistance to blood flow progressively increases. The blood eventually passes through minute arterioles which can expand and contract their diameter considerably and are responsible for controlling the exact quantity of blood required by the tissues. The blood then flows into thin-walled vessels called capillaries which service the tissue cells.

As Fig. 1.7 helps to illustrate, plasma, which is basically blood without the red cells, diffuses through the capillaries into the tissue spaces, taking in supplies of nutrients and oxygen (and, in the process, becoming known as 'tissue fluid'). Then it diffuses back into the other end of the capillaries, carrying away carbon dioxide and other waste products (the products of tissue activity) for disposal. Blood carrying these waste products then starts its return journey to the heart. It flows into minute veins (venules) and then into larger and larger veins until it eventually arrives back at the heart.

THE SYMPATHETIC NERVOUS SYSTEM

Basic blood pressure is controlled by the sympathetic nervous system (*see* Fig. 1.8). Sensors in the arteries, especially those in a little bulge (or 'body') in the carotid artery at the base of the neck, send impulses to their appropriate sympathetic centre. As a matter of interest, this small 'carotid body' is the place that practitioners of some martial arts squeeze to cause a sudden drop in the blood pressure in their opponents so that they lose consciousness. The pressure of the squeeze makes the sensors think that

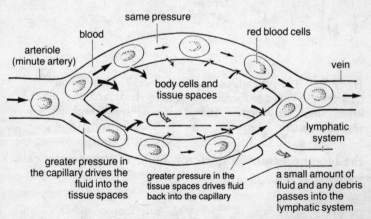

Figure 1.7 A larger view of capillary and tissue circulation

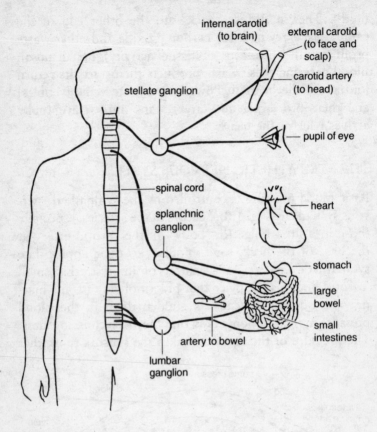

Figure 1.8 The sympathetic nervous system. The nerve centres (ganglia) are linked to specific organs in the body, and these are the organs which are adversely affected when the sympathetic nervous system is under pressure.

the blood pressure is much too high, so it is dramatically reduced.

MUSCLE PUMP

At this point, it is important to correct the popular myth that the circulation in the body is similar to that of a domestic radiator system. In a house, the central pump pushes the water round under pressure through the pipes to the radiators, where there is little resistance to the flow, then back to the pump where it is pumped out again, and so on. In the body, however, the circulation does not work in the same way. Although the heart pumps out blood through the arteries, it requires help to pump the blood back along the veins to the heart.

The heart exerts a great effort to push the blood through the arterioles, and by the time the blood reaches the small capillaries, which present considerable resistance to it, the force of the blood has only a minimum pressure left. Having started at a pressure of 120 units, it reaches the beginning of each capillary at the considerably lower pressure of 35 units.

This pressure is, however, higher than that of the tissue fluid (which is 15 units) so when blood arrives in the capillaries, the plasma in it is forced into the tissue spaces. By the time the plasma (now called tissue fluid) reaches halfway down a capillary, the pressure has dropped to around 10 or 15 units. However, the pressure of the tissue fluid is now greater than that of the blood, and this allows the tissue fluid to push back into the capillary again (*see* Fig. 1.7).

Blood leaves the capillary to enter the veins with a basic pressure of about 10 units. This is sufficient – along with the pumping effect of breathing and the constant rhythmic contractions of the vein walls, which pushes the blood along like a piston (in the same way that the intestines push food along) – to maintain the circulation when you

25

are lying down or sleeping. However, as soon as you start to move about, a new pumping force is needed.

When a person is active, large volumes of blood need to be returned to the heart, for, as we have already seen, the greater the level of activity, the greater the amount of blood needed to nourish the hard-working muscles. Gravity helps to drain areas which are above the level of the heart, but the main mechanism for returning the blood from the tissues is the muscle pump.

As the name suggests, muscles are at the centre of this pumping mechanism. When muscle relaxes, the tissue spaces and veins fill up with the fluid carried in by the arteries as, at rest, there is little force to return it to the heart. When a muscle contracts (see Fig. 1.9a & b), it drives the blood out of it and into the veins. Non-return valves in these veins ensure that the flow is in one direction only – towards the heart. Furthermore, a vital function of the muscle pump is that, as the contracting muscles expand, they also put pressure on adjacent tissues, which drives the tissue fluid out from these tissues back into the bloodstream. This action also compresses the veins, driving the blood in them back to the heart.

As we have seen, normal blood pressure is controlled by two main factors: the amount of blood that the heart is pumping out and the resistance of the capillaries. It also varies from person to person and according to the level of activity. When you are excited or exercising vigorously, your heart must pump at a higher speed to keep the pressure constant, since many more capillaries open up when more muscles are used. In a state of excitement or emergency, hormones are secreted by glands, which actually causes the blood pressure to rise. In both these situations, considerably more blood is needed to keep up the circulation, so reserves are called upon, causing your blood

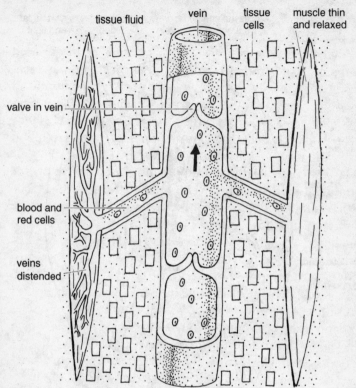

Figure 1.9a Muscle pump (muscle relaxed)

volume to rise. When you are sitting quietly or sleeping, there is less blood circulating and less pressure in the arteries.

CORONARY ARTERIES

Your heart is almost entirely made up of muscle known as the myocardium (from the Greek *muos*, 'muscle', and *kardia*, 'heart'). Like every muscle in your body, it needs a rich supply of blood, especially as unlike most other

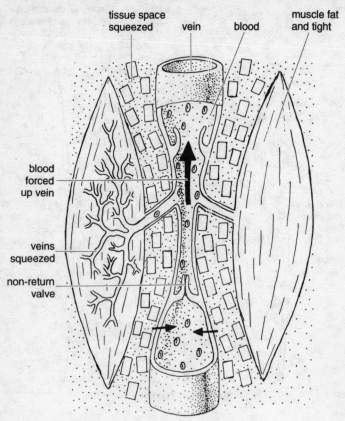

tissue space
squeezed

vein

blood

muscle fat
and tight

blood
forced
up vein

veins
squeezed

non-return
valve

Figure 1.9b Muscle pump (muscle contracted)

muscles, it has to work continuously throughout a person's life. It cannot utilize the blood being pumped around the inside of the heart; this blood is too far away from the muscle fibres to service them, and in any case, in half of the heart the blood is being pumped to the lungs and therefore contains little oxygen as it has just returned from supplying the body.

28

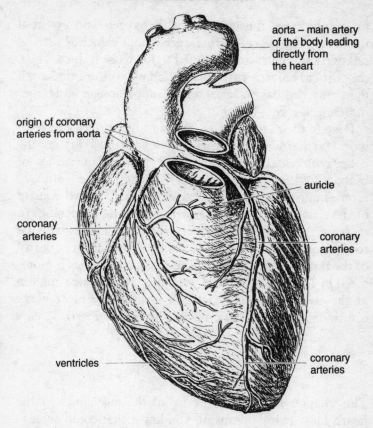

aorta – main artery
of the body leading
directly from
the heart

origin of coronary
arteries from aorta

auricle

coronary
arteries

coronary
arteries

ventricles

coronary
arteries

Figure 1.10   The heart, showing the coronary arteries

So the heart gets it own special supply of blood, through
the coronary arteries. This name is very descriptive: 'coronary' comes from the Latin word *corona*, 'crown' – and
these arteries encircle the heart just like a crown. As Fig.
1.10a shows, the two main arteries branch from the big
aorta almost immediately after the latter emerges from the
heart, and then divide into a network of smaller branches
covering the surface of the heart and running deep into it

to supply every muscle fibre with oxygen and essential nutrients. The heart – little larger than a clenched fist – is relatively small in size compared to the work it does. Thus, the coronary arteries are correspondingly shorter in length than most ordinary arteries which supply longer and larger muscles. (*see* Fig. 1.10.)

Despite their smaller size, the coronary arteries have to work far harder than other arteries in the body, as the heart requires such tremendously differing quantities of blood. To keep pace with these changes, the coronary arteries must be capable of extremely finely tuned control of the size of their inner diameter – dilating (widening) to increase the supply of blood to the heart and narrowing to decrease it (*see* Fig. 1.11a & b). This delicate control of the flow of blood through the coronary arteries is monitored by local reactions and overall by the stellate ganglion at the base of the neck, which is the uppermost nerve centre of the sympathetic nerve system (*see* Fig. 1.8).

The Silent Pump

This chapter began with praise of the mechanics of the heart. How many pumps do you know that could achieve such results? What's more, this powerful pump in your chest is able to circulate these huge quantities of fluid non-stop for up to a hundred years or more *and* quite silently – without even you being able to hear it. This is just as well, because if it were noisy, it would be like the alarm clock in the crocodile in *Peter Pan*, telling all our enemies exactly where we were! However, like all pieces of machinery, the heart does not always work properly. In the next chapter we will look at what can go wrong.

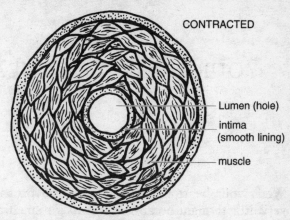

Figure 1.11a Constricted (narrowed) artery

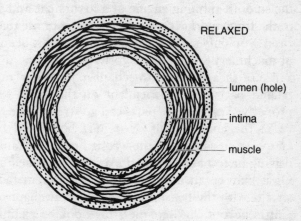

Figure 1.11b Dilated (widened) coronary artery

2

YOUR UNHEALTHY HEART

When your heart is working well, you probably give it very little thought because it does its job so efficiently. You could compare the heart and its control mechanisms to the smooth-running engine of a luxury car and your body to the framework. It's a rather sad fact of life that, in most cases, you only start to fully appreciate this beautiful piece of machinery when things go wrong.

A car is a complex mechanism that has many inter-related parts, each dependent on the other to function properly. Any of these parts can go wrong. The fault could be in the engine itself or it may be caused by outside factors such as putting the wrong fuel in the tank, reckless driving or too heavy a load exerting too much of a strain. Or it may be an amalgamation of different factors. And so it is with the heart and its control mechanisms.

It is beyond the scope of this book to examine all the possible causes of heart problems, but it is useful to look at the main things that can go wrong. First, we will look at the most common faults within the heart itself. Later, we will consider how other important influences such as diet and lack of exercise can cause or contribute to the poor functioning of the heart.

Faults Within the Heart

Broadly speaking, it is possible to sub-divide the internal faults into two groups of heart disease: chronic (*chronicos*='time', thus a disease that lasts over a period of time) and acute (*acutus*='sharp or pointed', a disease that produces sudden and severe symptoms).

CHRONIC HEART DISEASE

This is when your heart doesn't work as well as it should. There may be no symptoms for many years as the heart is able to compensate for a defect to an amazing extent. Its muscles often overdevelop, thus enlarging the whole heart, to cope with the extra workload. When the heart is no longer able to manage, one of two things may happen. There may be *congestive heart failure* – i.e. the heart is no longer able to pump the blood back to the heart as fast as it is being used so fluid begins to collect in the body, causing swelling of the ankles and other parts. Or it may be that the heart, suddenly unable to cope, fails rapidly, so that the series of events associated with congestive heart failure take place within days.

It is said that a doctor in Shropshire in the 1780s was told that the local healers gave patients foxglove leaves to chew for this problem. Being in no state to argue, the doctor tried them himself and then an infusion made from them on patients in heart failure. He was amazed how well this treatment worked. This is how the purple foxglove (or *Digitalis purpurea*) is supposed to have been discovered, and it (or, rather, its active ingredient) has remained the lynchpin of the treatment for congestive heart failure to the present day.

Among the main causes of chronic heart disease are:

- **Valve disorders**. The efficient pumping of the heart depends on four sets of non-return valves which ensure that blood flows in one direction only. Two valves allow blood into the two sides of the heart but prevent it returning into the veins when the heart pumps; the other two allow blood out of the heart into the arteries but prevent it from regurgitating as the heart fills. If a valve is not working properly – either through congenital deformations of the valve cusps (the flaps that open to let blood through) or through disease such as rheumatic fever, which distorts the valves – then, depending on the severity of the situation, the blood will leak back to some degree, and this will interfere with the normal pumping mechanism.

- **Diminishing elasticity of the arterial walls**. As we have seen, an artery is somewhat like an elastic balloon, expanding to absorb the surge of blood pumped by the heart throughout its branches and then gradually contracting until the next beat. This converts the pulsing of the heart output into a smooth steady supply of blood to the tissues. If the arteries lose their elasticity due to arterial disease, the fluid pushed through by heartbeat can only be accommodated if there is a significant rise in the pressure from each beat. This means that the person's blood pressure rises. The state of continued high blood pressure is known as hypertension (*hyper*='above'). As the heart makes more and more effort to pump out blood, it will, like all muscles in the body, increase in size to cope with the greater workload. However, there will come a point when it can develop no further and will thus begin to fail.

ACUTE HEART DISEASE

A heart attack is the general name for any sudden cessation of the normal function of the heart. The word 'function' is important. The heart often doesn't stop beating when it has an attack, but it *does* stop pumping effectively.

Under normal conditions, the muscles in the heart contract from the bottom up to diminish the size of the ventricles in a co-ordinated action thus achieving the maximum squeezing effect (*see* Fig. 1.6a). Immediately after it has contracted, a muscle fibre goes into a resting phase during which it cannot be stimulated, and it is then that the heart refills before the next contraction takes place. Immediately after a heart attack, the muscle contractions often go round and round the heart without any pattern at all because, by the time one wave has passed right round, the muscles have come out of the resting phase and can be stimulated again, so the contraction starts another futile round. Thus, the heart makes hundreds of mini-contractions, none of which do anything in the way of pumping. This is called ventricular fibrillation. As a result, blood does not get forced out of the heart to supply the heart muscles, the body or the brain.

IMPORTANCE OF RESUSCITATION

The brain is a very delicate instrument, and if it is deprived of blood for more than about four minutes, it is likely to suffer irreversable damage. Muscle is less vulnerable to an oxygen shortage, so the heart will survive much longer, continuing its futile contractions. Therefore, it is vital that a heart attack victim's blood be kept circulating through cardio-pulmonary resuscitation (CPR) – the 'kiss of life' and 'heart massage'. If this is done for long enough, oxygen will continue to reach the brain, preventing damage to it. The heart will often resume, or be made to resume, its proper function and the contractions will become adequate again. Indeed, it has been estimated that some 20,000 people die every year who could have been saved if someone present had known what to do at the time of the attack.

If you are with someone who appears to be having a heart attack, first summon help if this is at all possible. You only have about six mintues before the person's brain will be permanently damaged if no resuscitation measures are undertaken. Try to remember to look at the exact time that the patient became unconscious as this is valuable information to a resuscitation team. (*see* Appendix for instructions on cardio-pulmonary resuscitation.)

If the heart muscle is only deprived of blood for a short time, the person may make a complete recovery. More commonly, he or she will survive but with partial damage to the heart muscle. The temporary lack of oxygen will kill some of the muscle – hence the term *myocardial infarct*, which means 'death of heart muscle'. Although this damaged muscle will never recover, it is quite possible to live a perfectly healthy life without it as long as the remainder of the heart is fit and strong. In its prime, the heart muscle has enough power to allow you to run 100 metres in 10 seconds or so. Even when you are older and the heart muscle is not quite so fit, it still has considerable reserves of power. It is for this reason that, even with the death of some of the heart muscle, there is still plenty left for an average person to lead a normal life.

What causes a heart attack?

There are three main causes of heart attacks:

- blockage of the blood supply to the heart
- sudden disruption of the transmitting mechanism
- failure of the muscles through toxic interference

Blockage of the blood supply to the heart is the most common cause of heart attacks in middle to later life. This will be discussed at length in the next chapter, so only a brief summary will be given here. If the heart is suddenly deprived of its supply of blood, it will go into complete disarray. As we have seen in Chapter 1, the heart muscle gets its supply of blood via the coronary arteries. This supply can be diminished or even cut off completely if something goes wrong either with the coronary artery itself or with the mechanisms that control the internal diameter of the coronary artery. Although these arteries are relatively short compared to most arteries in the body, they have a tremendous amount of work to do in keeping pace with the heart's ever-changing fuel requirements.

The coronary arteries are capable of extremely delicate control of their internal diameters, dilating (widening) or narrowing them rapidly to increase or decrease the blood supply as necessary. This is very similar to an irrigation system. The water in large canals, drawing water from a river, flows into smaller and smaller canals until mere ditches supply the thirsty land. If there were no control over the flow, the canals nearest the source of the river would take all the water, leaving all the rest permanently dry. One way to overcome this would be to have an enormous river capable of supplying all the canals and ditches. In the body, there is not enough space for the huge quantity of blood that would be needed for such a large catchment area, so another method, which makes economic use of the fluid, has evolved.

This is similar to the manner in which the waters of the

Nile are controlled to make fertile the land on either side of the river for hundreds of miles. At times when a great deal of water is required in a particular area, either because it has become very parched or because some special activity such as planting is taking place, the main canal gates and those of the smaller canals supplying the area are all kept wide open. However, as soon as the area has received sufficient supplies, the gates begin to close, especially those of the little canals and ditches. In this way, the relatively meagre amount of water in the river can be regulated to supply all the requirements of a total land area hundreds of times larger than would have been possible without this elaborate control system.

However, as they are relatively small in diameter, this valuable property makes the coronary arteries particularly vulnerable. If they malfunction, even to a small degree, the supply of blood to the heart can be severely diminished (*see* Fig. 1.11a & b). If the artery is already narrowed through arterial disease, the supply may be closed off completely (*see* Fig. 3.2a & b).

Sudden disruption of the transmitting mechanism in the heart. This mechanism is responsible for the control and speed of the heartbeat. (*see* Chapter 1 for a full discussion of this.)

Toxic substances or infections can poison the heart muscle. The heart will continue working as long as possible, but when the effect reaches a critical point, heart failure is often almost instantaneous. Among the group of toxic substances that can do this are direct infections of the heart muscle such as by the flu virus, toxins from certain kinds of bacteria (which also cause some sore throats) and, of course, certain poisons. Infections can invade your body as a whole, attacking all your muscles including your heart. There is a real danger of inducing a fatal muscle failure if you take fairly vigorous exercise too soon after a viral infection, especially influenza. If your heart is still in an inflamed and sensitive state, it may not be strong enough to cope with the increase in workload, and it may suddenly go into uncontrolled contractions which could be fatal.

> Elizabeth, 23 and extremely fit, sadly died following a flu virus. She was on a skiing holiday with friends in Switzerland when she had an attack of flu. She stayed in bed for three days and took it easy for the next day. By the fifth day, she was so fed up with losing good skiing time that she went out with her friends on an advanced slope. On the way down, she suddenly fell and, when she eventually came to rest, remained motionless. When one of her friends reached her, she was already dead. A post-mortem found that her heart muscle and membranes were inflamed. This was attributed to the virus.

What else can cause problems?

There are many other factors which can interrupt the smooth running of the heart, especially an interruption of the oxygen supply to the lungs or a poison that prevents the blood from carrying it around. Severe loss of blood is another factor. However, this book is only concerned with those factors that affect the possibility of a heart attack. The main risk factors can be divided into those that can be controlled – unhealthy diet, lack of exercise, being overweight, smoking – and those that cannot be changed: age, heredity, sex, race, and national customs.

Controllable factors

Research has identified several areas of our lifestyles that contribute to heart problems. Preventative measures will be discussed in Chapter 6.

Unhealthy diet The main culprits in terms of affecting the heart are animal fat, sugar and salt. Eating excessive amounts of animal fat results in a build-up of fatty deposits in the walls of the arteries all over the body. These deposits can cause disease of the coronary arteries, adversely affecting the supply of blood to the heart. The utilization of fat in the body is balanced with the burning of sugar. Eating too much sugar upsets this balance, thus encouraging the development of fatty deposits in the arteries. This upsets the elasticity of the wall leading to high blood pressure. Excessive salt can also unfortunately lead to this.

During World War II, the food supply in Britain and Europe was only just adequate, but despite this, the governments managed to ensure that, with supplements and rationing, most people had a healthy balanced diet. This resulted in two things: overeating became extremely rare so few people were overweight; but even more important, extra fats in the form of fatty meat, butter, cream, margarine, rich sauces and puddings were in very short supply. Of course, many people were also much fitter during the war as so many were in the various armed forces or back-up services. As a consequence of all this, the incidence of coronary trouble dropped markedly as the war progressed, despite the obvious increase in stress which accompanied the era. It is noteworthy that the numbers of deaths due to heart disease increased again after the war as food supplies returned to pre-war levels. Of particular significance was the fact that this return of heart trouble came about at different times in different countries, coinciding with the relaxation of food rationing in each place.

Of course, the rationing of sugar also had a considerable effect on coronary disease, but as was explained earlier, since sugar metabolism and fat metabolism tend to be interrelated, the more balanced and moderate diet clearly had a considerable impact on the overall incidence of coronary disease.

It has also been noticed that certain cultures which have diets with less fat and sugar than Western ones also suffer less from coronary trouble. Notable among these are the Inuit (Eskimos) and the Japanese, whose traditional diets include large quantities of fish. However, coronary trouble is on the increase in Japan as the diet there becomes progressively more Westernized.

Alcohol, on the whole, does not have an adverse effect on the heart. Although, in larger amounts, it causes overall damage to the body, especially the brain and the liver, it has little effect on the vascular system. Indeed, as long as it is drunk in moderation, it tends to be a relaxant and can actually confer considerable protection against coronary attacks.

Medical papers have been published that imply that, because coffee makes people feel very tensed up and can increase their blood pressure, it increases the incidence of coronary thrombosis. However, a recent paper suggests that coffee improves the coronary circulation and thus actually reduces the risk. So – you pays your money and you takes your choice.

My own view is that coffee has a number of undesirable effects on a large number of people. It makes them very tensed up and have palpitations (when the heartbeat

41

becomes obvious). It can also be responsible for a chronic food allergy, so that after an initial boost from drinking a cup, the imbiber is afflicted with an overwhelming tiredness that can only be surmounted by another cup of the offending fluid; depression can also come about later and, on giving up the coffee, the person feels so much better in so many ways that they wished they had realized its effect years before. So, if in doubt, don't drink it!

Lack of exercise   If you take adequate exercise, this utilizes the heart muscle and keeps it at a high level of fitness. This ensures a good supply of blood through the coronary arteries and maintains the health of both these arteries and the heart muscle.

The amount of exercise you need to do largely depends on how much your body has become accustomed to taking. If you lead a very sedentary life and a brisk walk to the shop makes you a little breathless, this regular walk taken three times a week will confer almost as much protection as the regular circuit training of a professional footballer who has to run around the pitch 20 times before he gets out of breath. The rule is to take what is termed violent exercise, exercise enough to make you feel rather breathless on a minimum of three occasions every week.

Exercise is now fundamental to the recuperation of patients after heart attacks and to the future management of their heart disease. At one time, it was recommended that heart patients should take life at a very gentle pace, but, thankfully, this philosophy has now changed. Today, regular exercise is one of the most important factors both in helping prevent another attack and in increasing the prospects of survival in the unlucky event of one taking place.

I have vivid memories of my introduction to the new

philosophy that heart patients should be kept as fit as their hearts will allow instead of limiting their lives so that they become complete invalids on the grounds that the heart must not be stressed.

During World War II I was scheduled to meet an American general as he landed in England from the United States. As he stepped off the plane, I was alarmed to see that not only was he very out of breath but he also had very blue lips. After a quick feel of his pulse, the diagnosis of a coronary thrombosis was almost certain.

'You must sit down at once, sir,' I said, 'and remain quiet until I can get an ambulance to take you to hospital. I'm afraid that you will have to remain in bed for a long time.'

'Not at all, son,' he replied. 'I'm under the care of a Dr White in America, and he tells me to keep going and keep fit so that my heart will remain strong enough to overcome any attacks I may have in the future – this is my seventeenth.'

Needless to say, he made a good recovery, although today we would have looked after him very carefully for a few weeks until his heart had fully repaired itself after the attack. Only then would we have advised an exercise regime according to his capacity.

Being overweight Your heart is perfectly able to cope with a little extra weight. After all, many people can walk home with bags of heavy shopping without a great deal of effort. However, being overweight (obesity) is often caused by a poor diet and a lack of adequate exercise which, as we have seen above, is a cause of arterial disease.

Indeed, *losing* too much weight too quickly may be a strain on the system and lead to problems. The actor Peter Sellers, for example, had a bad thrombosis shortly after he had effected a massive weight loss. If you lose weight too rapidly, your body thinks that you have survived a bad famine. So, instead of a quite high percentage of the food that you take on board being unused, as is normal, everything is absorbed, turned into fat and stored as a precaution against the next famine. So an intake of food that would previously have caused you to lose or maintain your weight will now prove to be excessive, and you will put all the weight back on again and may even put on more.

Smoking This has been shown both to make it more likely that the coronary arteries will go into a spasm – which, of course, increases the actual chance of having a coronary attack – and to increase the incidence of arterial disease, thus making the effects of a coronary incident potentially more serious. Smoking can also cause chronic bronchitis and thus a poor exchange of oxygen and carbon dioxide in the lungs; the health of the heart muscle is then compromised by the lower oxygen content of the blood, and this may be a critical factor in determining the survival of someone who has a heart attack.

Stress This is commonly considered to be a factor in the onset of a coronary thrombosis, but I think that this is a misconception. By stimulating the sympathetic nervous system and thus dilating the coronary arteries, stress may actually be a positive factor in preventing a clot from blocking them. People with low sympathetic nervous activity – or low 'drive', as it is usually called – become very tensed up as the brain stimulates the anxiety centre (the only centre linking it to the sympathetic nerve system) to create a 'crisis' that will increase the output of adrenalin. This makes these people become very tensed up, and this is even more so in a stressful situation. Being more obvious, their stress may therefore seem to be contributary to any heart attack when, in fact, it is the low sympathetic 'drive' that is the basic cause.

In any event, coronary attacks often occur at 3 a.m. when a person is very relaxed and the 'stress' is turned off, allowing the artery to contract.

Factors that cannot be changed

There are certain risk factors that are impossible to change.

Age Your arteries tend to become more diseased as you get older. The most 'at-risk ages' are between 45 and 60 years.

Heredity A family history of heart problems – either congenital or acquired – increases the likelihood of trouble.

Sex Statistics show that more men than women suffer heart attacks. In recent years, the ratio is becoming more balanced, but the fact remains that men are more vulnerable than women. Every year, roughly 100,000 men and 70,000 women die from coronary heart disease in the British Isles. This is largely due to the female hormone oestrogen which offers the artery walls a considerable measure of protection from damage by fats, sugar, calcium and salt; it also helps women avoid the hardening of the peripheral arteries (i.e. those on the outer parts of the body) which causes a rise in blood pressure. In the UK 1400 females aged betwene 45 and 54 die of coronary attacks, but this soars to 7000 a year between the ages of

55 to 64 – after most women have reached the menopause and produce very little oestrogen.

This is one of the reasons why I am a firm believer in all women, if possible, being given HRT (hormone replacement therapy) when they arrive at the menopause. There is also the advantage that oestrogen stops calcium from being drawn out of the bones, causing osteoporosis (*osteo*='bone', *poros*='little holes'), which can lead to pain and broken bones. By keeping calcium in the bones where it belongs, HRT also prevents higher levels of calcium in the blood, which could settle into the arterial walls.

Race and national customs   There is a genetic factor that makes some races more prone to coronary trouble than others. For example, South Asians living in the UK have a 45 to 55 per cent greater chance of coronary heart disease than the indigenous population.

National customs – as has already been discussed in relation to the Japanese and Inuit – can have a considerable effect on the incidence of coronary disease. A very considerable campaign to promote better eating is thought to have caused, at least in part, a significant drop in deaths from coronary trouble in the United States. Other countries – including Britain – have instituted similar campaigns, but with less success.

This chapter has investigated some of the things that can go wrong with the heart and its control mechanisms. The next chapter will take a closer look at the main cause of heart attacks – an occlusion (blockage) of a coronary artery which interferes with the blood supply to the heart muscle – and will give a new insight into what actually causes the blockage.

3
WHAT CAUSES THE BLOCKAGE?

The most popular idea about what causes a blockage in the heart muscle's blood supply is that a clot forms in the artery completely blocking it, and that this clot comes about because of damage to the wall of the artery from pre-existing disease. More recently, a spasm of the coronary artery has been recognized as a factor in at least some cases. While accepting that the level of heart disease has a major bearing on the outcome of an attack, I hope to show that there is also a hitherto unrecognized factor which initiates the actual attack and without which the attack might never have taken place.

We will look in some detail at the four main events which can cause a blockage of this blood supply. In sequence, these are:

1 artery narrowed by its nerve control
2 artery narrowed by disease in its wall
3 arterial spasm further narrows or closes the hole in the artery
4 artery blocked by a clot

Artery Narrowed by Nerve Control

The sympathetic nerve chain is responsible for, among its many other functions, controlling the dilation and narrowing of the coronary arteries. It is one of three separate but interdependent nervous systems in the body. The other two are the central nervous system and the parasympathetic nervous system.

The central nervous system runs throughout the whole body and is the most important of the systems. It is dominated by the brain and includes all the ordinary sensory and motor nerves. It controls all voluntary actions and perceives all conscious sensations such as vision, taste and smell, hearing, skin sensations, muscle, joint and tendon status, and the pain of internal malfunctions such as injury or appendicitis.

The parasympathetic nervous system (*para*='beside'; *see* Fig. 3.1a) is also known as the 'vegetative system' as it mainly controls the digestive tract. When this nerve system is stimulated by the person eating, it causes secretion of digestive juices and the churning movements of the stomach and bowel. It mainly consists of a nerve centre in the brain and two long nerves (called the 'vagus' nerves, from the Latin for 'wandering') which meander all over the body on either side. The right and left vagus nerves supply most of the organs of the body and run parallel to the sympathetic nervous system. The parasympathetic works in opposition to the sympathetic, each balancing the other to maintain a harmonious balance.

The sympathetic nervous system: its name is derived from the French *sympathique* (which does not quite translate into the English 'sympathetic') because it was noticed that the heartbeat speeded up as a result of this nerve system being affected by emotion. The system influences

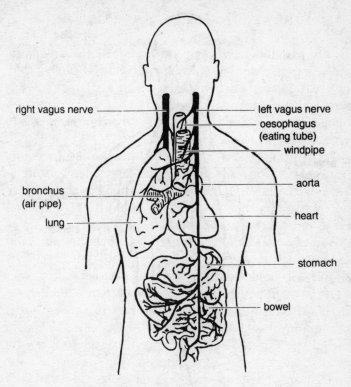

Figure 3.1a Vagus nerves (parasympathetic nervous system)

the running of the entire body and monitors and controls many parameters such as blood pressure, blood chemistry and repair. It comprises a chain of nerve centres (*ganglia*) connected by nerves to each other, to spinal nerves and to virtually every part of the body. As Fig. 3.1b shows, each nerve centre along the spine is linked to specific organs in the body, and it is the stellate ganglion which influences the supply of blood to the heart.

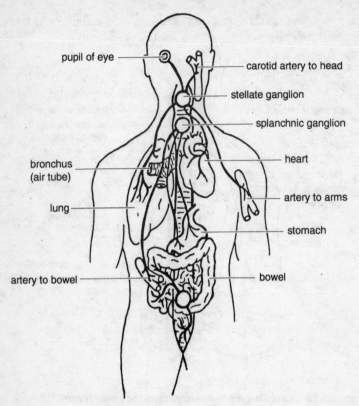

pupil of eye

carotid artery to head

stellate ganglion

splanchnic ganglion

heart

bronchus
(air tube)

artery to arms

lung

stomach

artery to bowel

bowel

Figure 3.1b Sympathetic nervous system

EMERGENCY RESPONSE

The sympathetic chain is also responsible for the body's
built-in response to emergency situations. In fact, it is part
of the adrenalin mechanism which is designed to put the
body into a state of efficiency in an emergency. In primitive
conditions, this kind of emergency would be a purely
physical one – an approaching lion or other dangerous
animal, perhaps. The sympathetic nervous system prepares

the body for instant and intense action – either fight or flight. As it does so, the person will experience:

- A rise in pulse and blood pressure.
- Trembling, which is actually small contractions of a number of muscles, to generate heat to increase body temperature. Everything works better at a higher operating temperature; think of reptiles which are very slow-moving if cold but can be very quick when heated by the sun.
- Sweating to prepare the skin for cooling during the supreme physical effort.
- An uncomfortable feeling in the stomach and a pallor of the skin as blood vessels contract to redirect blood from areas where it is not required to areas such as muscles and the brain where it may be urgently needed.
- Head and body hair standing on end (such as a lion's mane or cat's fur) as a (hopeful) protection against the teeth of the attacker and also as an aggressive postural effect to frighten off the enemy.
- Shedding of unnecessary weight, or at least the first stage of shedding it so that you feel sick and want to urinate and possibly defecate.
- Dilation of the pupils of the eye to let in more light.
- The sensation of fright.

Look at Fig. 3.1b again and you will see why these responses above would be experienced when the sympathetic nervous system is stimulated.

UPSETTING THE BALANCE

In a healthy body, the sympathetic nerve chain balances and opposes the parasympathetic. It is rather like a tug-of-war, with each nerve system balancing the other to maintain a state of harmony. If one side increases or decreases its output, the equilibrium is disturbed. If, under normal conditions, the sympathetic nerve system slows down, the parasympathetic responds by becoming more active. If one is stimulated, the other almost switches off. When, for example, the sympathetic is activated through fear, the parasympathetic almost completely cuts off its output so that energy-using processes – say, digestion – do not drain any energy during the crisis.

If the emergency lasts only a few minutes, as it would have done in the case of a prowling lion, this does not lead to problems. It is only when something causes a prolonged imbalance that any adverse effects are felt, and this can, of course, happen quite frequently in a modern environment. Say, under conditions of pressure, the digestive juices are turned off and the blood supply to the stomach is turned down to the barest minimum to conserve vital energy. This causes no problem over the short period of a primitive type of emergency, but when civilized stresses such as business, money or family worries arise, these tend to continue for days, weeks or months. This deprivation of the stomach may then cause trouble, even the development of a stomach ulcer. The problems caused by prolonged stress may also occur in other parts of the body.

ANGINA

As we have already seen, the stellate ganglion influences the size of the inner diameter of the coronary arteries. If the sympathetic share of the balance in the body is lowered, this diameter is maintained at a smaller size than normal (*see* Fig. 1.11a). As a result, the heart does not get quite the normal amount of oxygen. As the output of the sympathetic nervous system diminishes further, the diameter becomes increasingly smaller. In the early stages, this may have no noticeable effect; then, at a later date, it can give rise to what is known as angina-of-effort, which is felt as a sharp pain in the chest.

As a matter of interest, angina simply means 'pain'. You can have angina in other parts of your body. If you are suffering from one form of sore throat, for example, this is known as Vincent's angina. If the pain is felt in the chest, it is called angina pectoris (*pectoris*='chest').

Shortage of oxygen

Angina pectoris normally arises when a person takes some form of exercise or is particularly excited or anxious about something. In these circumstances, the heart works harder and the muscles require an increased supply of fresh blood. If the blood flow through the coronary arteries is diminished, the heart cannot get enough blood to supply its muscles with the required amount of oxygen. Like all muscles, the heart muscles become painful when short of oxygen, so the person experiences a fearful pain in the chest – and the arm.

Think of the pain of a cramp in your leg or even when your stomach is upset. The pain is very sharp indeed. In the case of your leg, the pain is actually felt in the muscle of, say, the calf involved. In the case of the heart, things are slightly different. I have already mentioned that, because of the huge amount of equipment that has to be packed into such a small space, many of our systems have to double up their functions. It was shown that, for instance, the muscles have to act as a pump to help transport the blood back to the heart as well as to enable you to move. In the same way, the nerves often supply more than one part of the body.

The heart shares a sensory nerve supply with the wall of the chest and down the left arm. Our hearts are almost always very strong and go many years without any problems, so if anything goes wrong, the brain assumes that it is the chest and/or the arm that are malfunctioning, not the reliable old war-horse in your chest. For this reason, the pain is felt as a vice-like sensation around the chest and down the arm, and not in the heart itself.

The pain experienced by a person during an angina attack usually goes after a few minutes' rest as the muscles recover, but it comes back again after another bout of exercise.

Keith, a 53-year-old barber, came to me complaining that he could only walk about 100 metres (330 ft) before he got a severe pain in the chest which he described as 'clamp-like' and when he found it difficult to breathe. After a rest, he was able to resume his walk until he had the pain again. He had been investigated and only a slight narrowing of his coronary arteries had been found. He was advised to continue with an artery-dilating drug, which gave him complete relief at the time.

However, the painful attacks had started up again and were becoming more frequent. Keith said he was getting worried and wanted my opinion. He said he also tired easily and had a lot of fibrositis between his shoulders

following a whiplash injury nine years previc
addition, he had been treated for a gastric ulcer son
before.

On examination, I was able to trace the root of the
problem. It lay in his spinal column and was causing an
upset in the sympathetic balance in his system, giving rise
to the angina and other health problems. After a total of
14 sessions of my form of physical medicine over a period
of 14 months, he has remained symptom-free for several
years. Keith also says that he has more energy, less digestive
trouble and feels far better in himself.

For Keith, angina pectoris was rather like an 'early warning' system that something was amiss in his body. Indeed,
the situation can get progressively worse until it reaches a
point where coronary arteries are too narrow to allow
a sufficient blood supply to nourish the muscles under
everyday working conditions.

Artery Narrowed by Disease in its Wall

All the arteries in the body, including the coronary arteries,
can be affected by atherosclerosis (*athere*='plaque',
skleros='harden') which is a disease in which plaque (a
deposit of fibrous material) forms in their walls. By press-
ing on the muscle and elastic tissue of the artery, the plaque
can damage and even kill it so that it is replaced by more
fibrous tissue. These degenerative changes actually occur
within the arterial wall, and fatty deposits start to appear
under the inner lining layer of the artery. These changes
can occur in any artery in the body and seldom cause
symptoms. It is virtually only in the coronary and cerebral
(brain) arteries that crises can occur. In the coronary arter-

ies, atherosclerosis causes heart attacks; in the cerebral arteries, it causes strokes. More than half of the artery can be closed off through atherosclerosis, which can block off almost all of the opening when the artery contracts (*see* Fig. 3.2a & b). This narrowing may not matter so much in a small artery, as it would not supply – or, therefore

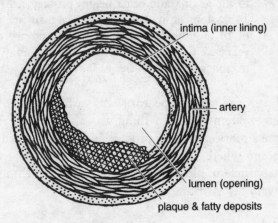

Figure 3.2a   Diseased arteries. Dilated artery

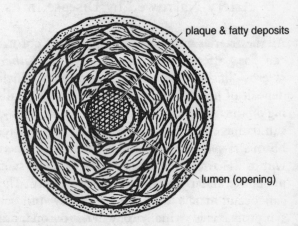

Figure 3.2b   Diseased arteries. Contracted artery

involve – a large volume of heart muscle. However, in a large artery, it would be likely to cause a major heart attack.

Atherosclerosis can interfere with the blood flow in several ways:

- The plaque and fatty deposits bulge into the artery (*see* Fig. 3.2b) and can cause a varying degree of difficulty in the passage of blood into the main heart muscle. This could give rise to angina-of-effort.

The plaque infiltrates and damages the lining of the artery. This may put the clotting mechanism into action. This clotting process is an essential part of your body's defences, designed to stop you bleeding to death. It is a complex system whereby, if your arterial system is punctured externally or internally, the hole can be plugged by the blood solidifying; chemicals in the body then activate the formation of string-like fibrous tisse (i.e. a clot) over the leak in an effort to seal it off. The centrepiece of the mechanism is the platelets in our blood.

Platelets are very small cells which, as their name suggests, are shaped liked plates. They act to limit the loss of blood by sticking to the tissues and to each other, forming a mound at, or very near, the site of a leak. This adhesion, helped by other local reactions, rapidly starts to form a local clot which slows up or even blocks the leakage of blood through the artery wall.

However, sometimes, the platelets can act without the artery wall having been punctured. In a normal course of events, the walls of an undamaged artery are lined with such a smooth membrane that the platelets cannot stick to it, and the blood flows through without interruption. When an artery becomes diseased, however, the fatty deposits in the wall cause the smooth lining to bulge inwards and become rough. As soon as the platelets in the blood come into contact with these patches of damage, they stick to it and to each other and form a local seal. This can gradually extend and may block the whole vessel.

- The fatty deposits can press so hard on the blood vessels in the actual wall of the artery that they burst. This bleeding within the arterial wall may further damage the already diseased lining of the artery and may also increase the swelling into the channel.

- Such injuries in the artery tend to 'calcify' as the fatty element reacts with calcium in the blood. This is not dissimilar to the way scum forms when the calcium impurities in water react with the fat of the soap to produce this hard insoluble product.

- The calcified plaques in the artery walls replace the numerous elastic fibres, so reducing its flexibility. This means the artery wall cannot expand in the normal manner to take up the wave of pressure from the heart's contraction and then push the blood smoothly and evenly into the heart muscle.

As the disease progresses in the arterial wall, the diameter of the artery becomes smaller and smaller here and there. The first symptoms can be felt as angina-of-effort. This is the result of a lack of oxygen in the heart muscle due to less blood passing to the heart, and can give rise to a pain in the chest usually during exercise. The affected person is usually able to walk a definite distance before the pain starts, and this distance remains quite constant for that individual.

Increased narrowing, especially if accompanied by the presence of fibrous tissue (which develops after the death of muscle in the artery wall) from previous trouble, can cause more sinister problems. The person, seriously crippled on activity, will need to have this constriction forced open or else a bypass operation, in which a vein in the leg is inserted in place of a damaged coronary artery. More serious still is a sudden accumulation of blood platelets on the diseased wall, which can cause a rapid and total obstruction of the artery resulting in a massive heart attack.

CAUSES OF ATHEROSCLEROSIS

Atherosclerosis is believed to start in childhood and develop slowly through life. The cause is still not fully known but research has discovered that there is probably not a single cause but a number of factors which increase the likelihood that these fatty deposits will develop on the arterial wall. The main ones are: high blood cholesterol levels, high blood pressure, smoking and diabetes. This section looks at how these risk factors contribute to the build-up of arterial disease.

High blood cholesterol levels   Cholesterol is probably one of the most talked about, and least understood, of the body's chemicals. It has had rather a 'bad press' in terms of heart disease, but it is only when there are excess amounts in the body that it may form deposits in the arterial wall. Indeed, when kept within normal limits this much maligned chemical is so important to our good health that you may be interested to know more about it.

Cholesterol is a fatty substance which is found in the blood and manufactured naturally in the body by the liver, bowel and many other cells. It is a vital raw material for a number of things. It is an essential component of the plasma membranes which are the outer linings of the body's cells, separating the cell structures from the tissue fluids. It is also a basic constituent of the bile salts, which are necessary to help break up fats during digestion.

But possibly its most important role is the part it plays as one of the raw materials of the huge range of equally misunderstood chemical messengers, or hormones, in the body, grouped under the name of steroids. There are three main types of steroids:

- **Testosterone** stimulates growth during puberty in boys and also the synthesis (building) of proteins. It maintains the male sexual organs and is responsible for the male secondary sexual characteristics. Athletes illegally trying to build up their muscles for enhanced performance usually take testosterone or one of its close relatives.

- **Oestrogen** stimulates growth of the secondary sex organs during puberty in girls. It also maintains the female sex organs and is responsible for the female secondary sexual characteristics. As we have seen, it also retards calcium-loss from bone and, in this way, protects women from heart disease.

- **Cortisone** is a hormone secreted by the cortex (outer layer) of the adrenal glands. An old-fashioned term for these are the suprarenal glands, which describes exactly where they are located: *supra*='above', *renal*= 'kidney'. Cortisone is also, by a strange coincidence, a misunderstood and much maligned substance. Many patients are afraid of this substance when it is given as a drug because they have heard so many adverse tales about it: however, used properly, it can be extremely beneficial. Criticism of any possible side-effects must, in any event, be considered against the alternative of not giving the person cortisone.

Cortisone has a number of effects upon the body. Most importantly, it speeds up the breakdown of proteins, increases the vaso-constriction effect (i.e. closing down, especially of arterioles) in the presence of either inflammation or allergy, and it is also a powerful inhibitor of the inflammatory reaction iself. It was discovered when the phenomenon of pregnant women suddenly undergoing a dramatic improvement in their arthritic condition was investigated; they were found to have an unusually high level of cortisone in their blood. When cortisone was given to patients crippled with arthritis, it resulted in a dramatic improvement. Where once people went blind in their hundreds with an inflammation of the iris of the eye, those with this condition now run little or no risk of losing their sight – because of the administration of cortisone. My last example, although there are many more, is of the disease poly-myalgia. Many muscles and joints become painfully inflamed for over a year. Although the disease even-tualy burns itself out, it can leave painful permanent damage behind. However, cortisone, if given through the active phase, will protect the patient so that, as the disease vanishes and the cortisone is discontinued, he or she is left – after a reasonably pain-free disease – with no after-effects at all.

Properly used, cortisone is a wonderful drug. My mother, when in her 70s, became a respiratory cripple after an attack of pneumonia and could hardly cross the hospital ward without becoming totally out of breath. After taking cortisone she was able to resume a near normal life.

Unfortunately, the drug is rather like an expensive sports car which has vivid acceleration to pull it out of trouble, excellent brakes to match and superb roadholding to cope with the considerable top speed. Such a car may be one of the most controllable and safest on the road – but put it into the hands of an 18-year-old lunatic who drives it at 120 mph through rush-hour traffic and people will start to scream that such a dangerous vehicle should be forbidden on the roads. Similarly, cortisone, such a powerful and useful weapon, is capable of sad abuse.

Cholesterol levels in the blood are influenced by several factors, the most important of which is diet. The blood cholesterol level is associated with the amount and type of fats in your diet. Cholesterol is carried in the blood in the form of lipoproteins which are water-soluble complexes of fat and protein. There are various types of lipoproteins including those designated HDL (high-density lipoproteins) and LDL (low-density lipoproteins). LDL carry cholesterol to the tissues, thus increasing deposits in arteries, whereas HDL, which is found in 'saturated' animal fats, takes cholesterol from cells and promotes its removal by secretion by the liver in the bile.

It is important to eat a diet that has the correct ratio of LDL and HDL to maintain a suitable level of blood cholestrol. A diet which is high in LDL can be a significant cause of arterial disease, whereas a diet which has a higher ratio of HDL can protect the arteries and actually reverse the damage, at least to some extent. It is interesting to note that exercise is also believed to raise HDL levels in the blood. Cholesterol itself is found in abundance in animal fats and egg yolks, but eating cholesterol will not signif-antly raise blood cholesterol levels.

High blood pressure eventually leads to atherosclerosis. However, raised blood pressure often goes unnoticed until it has caused significant damage. The most important symptom of high blood pressure is that there are no symp-toms, at least not until a very late stage. It is vital that everyone have their blood pressure checked regularly, so that any increase can be discovered early enough for it to be controlled and any damage prevented. Symptoms that arise later on can be tiredness, headaches and palpitations.

Smoking upsets the ratio of HDL and LDL and so has a significant effect on the degree of damage that takes place in the coronary artery wall. This, in turn, increases the severity of a heart attack if this takes place. Published medical papers generally agree that, if a person smokes under 20 cigarettes a day, they have a moderate increase in the probability of a heart attack; 20 or so cigarettes a day doubles the risk; and many more cigarettes than this actually increases smokers' chances of a coronary by four times over non-smokers. This is one of the few fields in which nature has been kind: if you stop smoking, the changes are largely reversible, so that after a year or two the risk would be no more than that found in someone who had never smoked.

Diabetes upsets the enzymes in your body and increases the tendency towards arterial disease. Indeed, arterial dis-ease can become so bad in a person with diabetes that all the arteries in the body are vulnerable to thrombosis. However, if it is diagnosed at an early stage, diabetes can almost always be controlled. I feel very strongly that everyone should have their urine and blood pressure checked at regular intervals, especially as they approach their 40s and are therefore more prone to coronary attacks.

Arterial Spasm Further Narrows or Closes the Hole in the Artery

We have already seen that a low level of imbalance of the nerve control to the coronary arteries will result in a modest, continuous narrowing of the vessel wall. Under extra heart output during exercise, this may cause the pain of angina because the muscle is not getting sufficient oxygen. An increased sympathetic imbalance can reach such a point that the artery goes into a spasm, closing it partially or completely; this will cut off the blood supply to the heart muscle, causing an attack similar to a thrombosis. One of three things will result:

- the artery may reopen reasonably rapidly before any damage to the heart muscle takes place and the patient will recover completely.
- the artery remains in spasm and the patient could die with no clot present.
- when the artery is in a spasm, a clot forms at the site of arterial disease and this will block off the artery semi-permanently, resulting in the death of the muscle supplied by the artery.

The effects of the spasm are obviously much more serious in a diseased artery, as it is already narrowed and it will be easier for the spasm to close down the opening. The blockage of the flow of blood – combined with the loss, because of the disease, of the special smooth lining that prevents clotting – will readily result in a thrombus (clot) forming, leading to a heart attack. If the patient survives, the heart muscle that has actually died will gradually form into fibrous tissue to keep the heart wall intact. This 'patch' can sometimes slowly start to bulge under the pressure of the blood in the ventricle at each contraction, and occasionally such scar tissue actually bursts, leading to the death of the patient.

Artery Blocked by a Clot

Clots can get into the coronary system and lodge in an artery, thus blocking it. However, this is very rare. There are few sources of such clots, since all the blood from the body goes through the lungs, which act as a very fine filter. Therefore the clot has to come from somewhere beyond the lungs. There are two possibilities: it either breaks off from a diseased valve, or it breaks off from a clot on the wall of a damaged larger coronary artery and blocks a smaller branch further down. Neither of these is very common.

The Severity of a Heart Attack

A heart attack caused by blockage of blood to the heart muscle can range from being so minor that no symptoms are felt, to a massive attack that is fatal. The seriousness of the episode depends on five main factors:

- *The actual site of the blockage*. The nearer to the beginning of the artery the blockage occurs, the more of the heart muscle is involved and the more serious is the attack. Arteries in the body are rather like trees. They start with a main supply like the trunk of a tree and then divide into smaller and smaller branches. The larger the artery, the greater the volume of heart muscle that will be served by it and thus damaged. Fortunately, blockage usually occurs in one of the branches quite a way down, so only around one fifth of the actual heart muscle has its supply of blood cut off or dramatically reduced.

- *The completeness of the blockage.*
- *The speed of occlusion (blockage).* If the blockage has been caused by a slowly increasing obstruction, other nearby arteries in the heart will have been able, over time, to compensate by supplying the heart with an ever-increasing 'collateral circulation' (a parallel circulation that sends branches into a site that has a restricted supply). The effect of the final obstruction will then be much less, as the muscle will continue to be supplied to some extent by this alternative circulation.
- *The type of obstruction.* If it is a spasm, it may relax leaving no after-effects.
- *The degree of the person's activity at the time of the attack.* When a person is lying in bed, the heart is reasonably rested and there are few waste products present. If the same person were playing squash, there would already be many waste products in the heart. In this situation, if the muscle is cut off from its blood supply there would be a critical shortage of oxygen in a much shorter space of time. Therefore, the chance of a massive death of the heart muscle is very much greater if the blockage occurs when a person is exercising vigorously.

More about the Spasm

This chapter has established the importance of a spasm of
the coronary artery as a cause of the crisis which leads to
arterial blockage. We have seen that arterial disease has
an important influence on the severity of a blockage: a
spasm of an undamaged artery may not close it down
completely and a clot may not form; the additional narrowing by disease can make the attack fatal. However,
arterial disease alone is seldom the culprit. The answer
lies with the all-important causes of the spasm. Through
an analysis of this subject, the next chapter reveals a whole
new approach to the topic.

4

WHAT CAUSES THE SPASM?

If coronary attacks are largely caused by a spasm of a coronary artery, it follows that the next point we need to look at is what causes that spasm. In this chapter, I shall explain how the spasm is triggered by a malfunction of the stellate ganglion – the group of ganglia, or 'little brains', that lie at the base of the neck. The ganglia, which are part of the sympathetic nerve chain, have the vital function of the overall control of the flow of blood through the coronary arteries.

What causes the stellate ganglion to malfunction? The answer lies in your spinal column. In my experience, the fundamental cause of many coronary attacks is an old injury which has jolted or twisted the upper part of the back giving rise to serious repercussions throughout the whole body. Readers of my first book, *The Back and Beyond*, will be familiar with this theory, but at this point, I would like, in the words of Dylan Thomas, 'to begin at the beginning' and recap on the main points.

The Spinal Column

If problems in your back can be directly associated with coronary attacks, it is important to understand its anatomy and functions. Your spine supports your body, but it is also flexible enough to allow you to move in various directions – to stand up, sit down, twist, bend and stretch. As Figs. 4.1a & b show, this flexibility is brought about by the separation of the vertebrae by elastic discs which allow movement between each individual vertebra.

A complex system of little joints, called 'facet joints', helps to stabilize the back and keep any movement within sensible limits (see Fig. 4.2). This is complemented by a widespread network of primitive wire-like bands of fibrous tissue called ligaments (see Fig. 4.3). These criss-cross all the joints in the body and help both to stabilize the joints and limit excessive, damaging movement.

Running along the length of the spinal column is a complex system of bundles of muscles (see Fig. 4.4). These muscles, which are, of course, controlled by the motor centre of the brain, are the source of power for the spine's movement and also maintain your posture when you are sitting or standing still. As we have seen in Chapter 1, the muscles also play a vital role in the flow of blood back to the heart from the tissues, where it is at almost zero pressure. Fig. 1.9b shows that, when a muscle contracts, this has the effect of compressing both it and the surrounding tissues, thus squeezing the blood out of them so that it travels into and up the veins. Special non-return valves ensure that the blood flows only towards the heart.

In fulfilling its function of returning blood from themselves to the heart, the muscles – collectively the muscle pump – play a role which is central to my theory. When the muscle fibres are relaxed, the veins and tissue spaces fill with, respectively, plasma and tissue fluid. As the muscle fibres contract, they compress the veins and tissue spaces thus forcing all this fluid back into the bloodstream. When everything is working well, there is always an

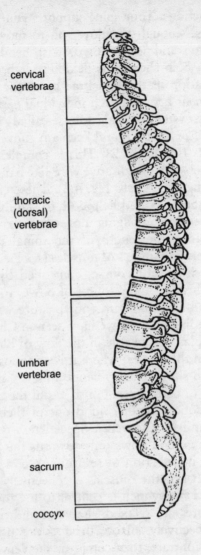

cervical
vertebrae

thoracic
(dorsal)
vertebrae

lumbar
vertebrae

sacrum

coccyx

Figure 4.1a These are the divisions of the spine.

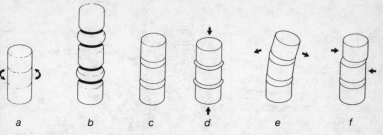

Figure 4.1b The mechanical function of the discs. In diagram *a*, flat surface against flat surface allows only rotational movement; *b* and *c* show these surfaces with an added layer of elastic tissue (the intervertebral discs), permitting all kind of movement; *d* shows compression, and *e* and *f* illustrate backwards, forwards, side to side, and sliding motions

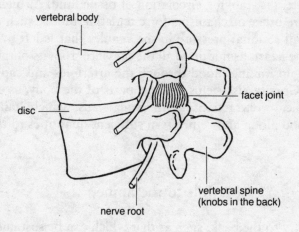

Figure 4.2 A normal facet joint

adequate return of blood from the tissues to the heart. During the daytime, the muscles are usually constantly active, performing all the movements of a healthy back; therefore, they are also pumping and ensuring an

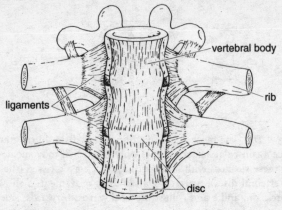

Figure 4.3 Ligaments

adequate, fast-moving circulation of tissue fluid. At night, there are other mechanisms for circulating blood, such as the small residual pressure in the venules that is left over from the heart, as not quite all the pressure from its output is used up forcing blood through the arterioles and capillaries. Gravity also helps in some parts of the body, as do rhythmical contractions of the vein walls, which 'milk' the blood along and return it in suffcient quantities to the heart.

A Jolt to the Spine

An injury to the back, such as that which can be sustained in a car accident, when falling down stairs or slipping on a floor, can interfere with the pumping mechanism. Such an injury bruises the delicate little facet joints which stabilize the back. The muscles across the joint react to the situation by going into a powerful contraction, or spasm, to protect the joints. This spasm is nature's way of putting

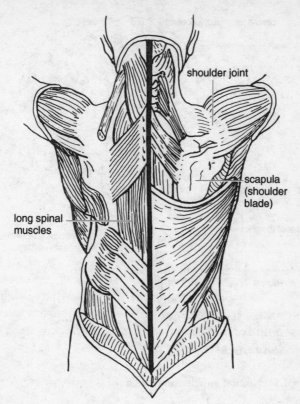

Figure 4.4 Spinal Muscles

the injured area into a restrictive corset or splint to limit the movement of the associated vertebrae and give the joints time to rest and repair themselves. Being a normal contraction of a muscle – although initiated by impulses not from the brain (*see* Fig. 4.5) but from the damaged joint (*see* Fig. 4.6) – it does not produce any symptoms and so the person remains unaware of its presence.

Unfortunately, due to the mechanics of the spine, the plan backfires. In the first place, the spasm of the muscles

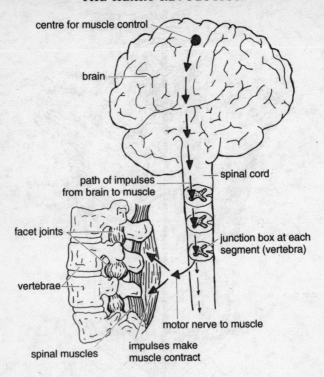

Figure 4.5 Normal muscle contraction

does very little to limit the movement between the vertebrae, and, second, the facet joints are actually put under extra pressure as the spasm pulls the vertebrae together. The injury to the joints is maintained or is made even worse, and nature responds by maintaining the spasm – so the situation is never alleviated. When muscles are in spasm and thus tight all the time, they are obviously not capable of pumping efficiently, so fluid tends to accumulate in the area involved. As the excess fluid – oedema – builds up, it eventually leads to serious waterlogging in the affected area (*see* Fig. 4.7).

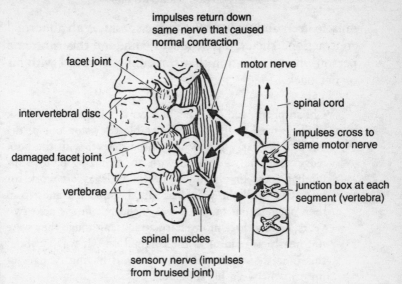

Figure 4.6 Contraction of a muscle spasm

Build-up of Congestion

The person may remain symptom-free for many years. There may be enough movement of the back, combined with the other forces that return the blood to the heart (i.e. gravity and the residual pressure in the veins) to maintain a very slow-moving circulation. However, the effects are cumulative: the muscles and nearby tissues will be suffering from the increasing lack of oxygen-rich blood and the build-up of waste products in the oedema.

As time goes on, this 'traffic jam' gets progressively worse as the joints further deteriorate and the protective spasm increases. Finally, the condition becomes so bad that it reaches a critical point when – due to lack of oxygen and the build-up of waste products – the muscle protests by going into a cramp. This cramp is generated in the muscle itself and, in contrast to the spasm, is an abnormal contraction. The cramp produces pain, and this is often a person's first realization that something is wrong with his or her back.

> Christopher, aged 31, had had no trouble with his back until he tried to lift a semi-portable television out of the boot of his car. He had just raised it level with the boot ledge when he was seized with an agonizing pain in his lumbar spine (in the lower back). He was off work for two days until the pain had largely subsided and, from then on, felt that his back was 'delicate'. In the next two years, he had three more sharp attacks, although they were not nearly as painful as the original one. It was at about this time that he noticed that he was having twinges of fibrositis between his shoulders.
>
> He came to see me as, despite having had various treatments, he was concerned that his back felt 'vulnerable' and the frequency of the attacks was increasing. On being questioned, he admitted that he had been getting very tired, possibly for about a year, and that he was also under treatment for a stomach problem. He said that he had been becoming very tensed up for some while and recently had had minor depression. He had been a keen rugby player until his late teens and remembered at least two occasions in the scrum when he had had really painful compressional jolts to his spine.

Another common way that trouble in the thoracic (chest) part of the back is noticed can be demonstrated in this story told by Alice, aged 43, who came to see me with a bad pain in her left arm.

> Alice had fallen off her horse about 20 years previously. She had been winded and a bit shaken at the time, but

managed to remount and finish her ride. She had rapidly got over the bruising and had forgotten about the episode – until I had asked.

About six years before she came to see me, she had begun to have slight discomfort and even a slight ache between her shoulders after sitting typing or reading for any length of time. Four months ago, she suffered a bad pain in her left arm which, although it varied a great deal, had never really gone away. A particularly bad bout had brought her to see me. She confessed to having a lot of headaches, and related both these and the pain to tension. She was beginning to tire easily and generally did not feel very well.

Affect on Adjacent Tissues

Long before the effects of the diminished muscle pump have reached this critical point, the waterlogging will have started to spread and affect adjacent tissues in the catchment area, which also depend on the squeezing action of the muscles (*see* Fig. 4.7a & b). In the context of this book, one of the most important of these nearby tissues is the sympathetic nerve chain which lies close to the spinal muscles in the lower neck and upper thoracic part of the spine.

As discussed in Chapter 3, this chain of nerve centres is one of three interdependent nerve systems in the body. It is made up of 'computers' which influence the running of the body machine and monitor and control a vast number of things such as blood pressure, blood chemistry and repair. It is also part of the adrenalin mechanism, in which the chemical messengers have a similar effect as the sympathetic system itself, and are also responsible for the body's built-in response to emergency situations.

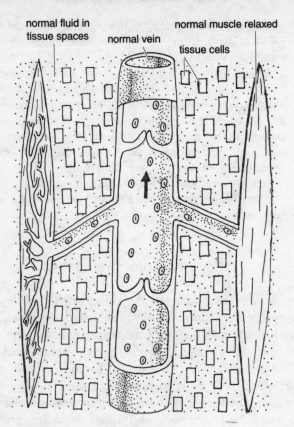

Figure 4.7a Normal muscle contraction

In Chapter 3, we saw that the sympathetic nervous system works in harmony with the parasympathetic, each pulling against the other in a 'tug-of-war' to maintain equilibrium. If one 'team' weakens its pull, the other becomes correspondingly more dominant. If one 'team' become extra-active, the other's influence lessens considerably. So in a situation where oedema causes a lessening of the sympathetic pull, the parasympathetic will have a

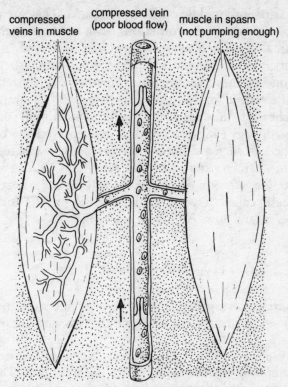

Figure 4.7b Muscle spasm resulting in oedema (excessive tissue fluid)

stronger influence than normal in the area supplied by the affected sympathetic ganglia.

The controlling centre of the parasympathetic nervous system is in the brain stem; this is surrounded by the skull so it is well protected and is unlikely to be upset by outside influences. In fact, it rarely malfunctions. Nature has not been so kind to the sympathetic chain, however. Its nerve centres, and they are numerous, lie near the muscles of the back, mainly in the chest area but also in the mid-lumbar region (middle of the lower back). They are prone to upset from adverse conditions, such as waterlogging, in the area. If all the nerve centres are depressed in their activity, then all sympathetic activity will diminish.

If one or more centres of sympathetic drive, or tone, are affected, it follows that the corresponding branch or branches of the parasympathetic system will be less opposed, thus exaggerating their influence on the organs supplied. In such a situation, the person will start to show certain characteristic signs and symptoms of a new syndrome (i.e. a group of symptoms and signs that make up a disease) called 'hyposympathetic tone', or HST for short (*Hypo* means 'low' or 'below normal'.)

HypoSympathetic Tone

HST affects a surprisingly large number of people and can, when severe, cause considerable distress and incapacity.

> Pauline, a 30-year-old secretary, came to see me with fibrositis between her shoulders and in her neck. The pain was becoming worse and she felt she needed help. It had started to radiate down her left shoulder and arm, and during particularly bad episodes, it went down into her left hand affecting her middle, ring and little fingers. On being questioned, she said she had been twice to see a hospital consultant because of her excessive tiredness. She had actually been referred to him by another consultant who was treating her for indigestion. She also experienced dizzy spells if she suddenly stood up, and had bad headaches over the left side of her head. She was very tense, and the previous year had seen a psychiatrist about a depression.
>
> On examination, Pauline showed a marked curve in the

chest part of her spine, her blood pressure was on the low side and her stomach was very tender. She had considerable limitation of movement in her neck and there was spasm of the spinal muscles, from her skull (where the muscles were tender) to the low thoracic spine. Pauline showed all the signs and symptoms of HST. However, after 11 treatments to her spine, the thoracic area became much looser and she gradually lost all her symptoms.

Many people who come to me, like Pauline, say that no one had previously been able to co-ordinate their symptoms. However, the signs of HST are so obvious that it can be readily diagnosed and successfully treated. The symptoms fall into four main categories:

- effects of low sympathetic drive
- effects of parasympathetic overactivity
- compensatory reactions of the brain
- thoracic and lower neck trouble.

Let us look at each of these symptom groups in more detail.

EFFECTS OF LOW SYMPATHETIC DRIVE

Tiredness that can be extreme and apparently unaccountable is usually the first and only symptom for several years. After a time, affected people feel not only tired but also unwell. Sometimes they can become seriously ill.

Tiredness caused by low sympathetic drive has certain distinct characteristics. It seems to peak at around 3.00 or 4.00 in the afternoon, after which the person usually perks up again. Sufferers also tend to 'flake out' completely when they get home from work, but soon revive after a short rest. Indeed, they often say that a five- or ten-minute rest or sleep is a good pick-me-up for excessive tiredness at any time of day.

Restful holidays are often recommended to sufferers, but they are not a great success for anyone with HST. If the person is to feel as well as possible the sympathetic nervous system needs a challenge to maintain a reasonable level of drive, and a holiday that simply involves lying about seldom does that. Even if apparently benefited, the person seems to go right back to square one a few weeks after returning and might just as well not have gone away.

Arthur, aged 48, was a director in a firm of stockbrokers. He had been feeling under par for several years, but nothing abnormal had been found in his annual medical check-up. In fact, he had been complimented and reassured because his blood pressure was a little on the low side.

A year before he came to see me, he had experienced a bad pain in his chest when out for a walk. His heart had been fully investigated but had showed no abnormalities when he was in hospital. Two months before we met, he had had a second similar attack and had once again been fully investigated, with no positive result. It had eventually been decided that the cause of his problem was the excessive stress he had been living under, and so he had been advised to go on a relaxing holiday. He had gone on a Mediterranean beach holiday for three weeks, during which he had felt a great deal worse and, on returning home, had been referred to me.

He had considerable tell-tale spasm of the thoracic chest muscles, and told me he had been suffering from mild indigestion for a number of years. The relaxing holiday had further lowered his sympathetic drive, which needs a certain amount of stress and tension to increase its output, and for that reason he felt so much worse. Treatment to the chest and spine soon had him back to normal.

Low blood sugar (hypoglycaemia) is another symptom of low sympathetic drive. People may have sudden 'hypo' attack which make them feel weak and cold, sometimes with a clammy sweat. They may also experience a sense of unease, even a feeling of impending doom.

Low blood pressure is also a common sign. In most cases, it is very much at the lower end of what is usually regarded as normal. Sufferers often say that their blood pressure has been rather low for a number of years, but they were not aware that it was a problem. Common effects of low blood pressure are dizzy spells and a faint feeling when you stand up suddenly, especially after lying down. If someone is in late middle age and has had the problem for many years, their blood pressure often begins to rise slowly to well above normal for their age. After a period of fluctuation, it then remains high and the level is often such that it requires treatment to bring it back to a safe figure.

EFFECTS OF PARASYMPATHETIC OVERACTIVITY

Indigestion in some form is a very common symptom of HST. The activity of the parasympathetic nervous system causes the secretion of a high level of acid which inflames the stomach lining, making it extremely sensitive. This may show itself in a fairly mild way. Often people say that they cannot stop nibbling, which is nature's way of mopping up excess acid. Some sufferers lose their appetite as the stomach behaves as if it resents food being put into it; they may also complain of frequent belching. Many of my patients insist that they are bringing up air – but it is actually a subsconscious swallowing of air in an effort to separate the sensitive walls of the stomach.

If the condition deteriorates, there may be indigestion with such symptoms as a feeling of a leaden weight or pain in the stomach. In extreme circumstances, a gastric (stomach) or duodenal (beginning of the small bowel) ulcer may result.

Allergic reactions may occur as the inflamed stomach becomes unusually sensitive to irritating foods. If this happens, it will sometimes activate the body's early warning system which enables tissues to recognize a minute trace of a substance that has caused trouble previously.

An allergy is a normal reaction to an irritation, taken to a completely abnormal level. Imagine that a police car sees a red Rover being driven so dangerously that it is swerving all over the motorway. This information is put into the 'action memory' of the police force. Other cars such as Fords, BMWs and Vauxhalls go by but they are not noticed by the squad. Suddenly, another red Rover is seen and immediately the avenging police swoop. Patrol cars block both carriageways of the motoroway and its approach roads. Everything comes to a standstill: traffic cannot move, hungry motorists cannot get near to the service station and no repair teams can attend to any problems on the road itself.

For the police to converge on a possible offender is a normal reaction and it may well result in the apprehension of a dangerous driver for the good of all. However, as with an allergy, when this response to a situation (or substance) that is seen as harmful is taken to such extremes, it can result in chaos.

Allergic reactions to certain food substances usually regress as the stomach improves with treatment to the protective spasm in the back muscles. Occasionally, however, they need treatment in their own right.

COMPENSATORY REACTIONS OF THE BRAIN

Tension is often a dominant symptom of HST. Many sufferers do not realize quite how tensed up they are feeling until they have been treated.

Depression has many causes, but can also be one of the symptoms of HST. Sadly, if the person has a depressive personality, or even if he or she has no apparent worries, this tensed-up state can lead to attacks of depression which may be serious enough to necessitate a consultation with a psychiatrist.

This tense state of mind is actually a mild version of fright generated by the brain to boost the output of the sympathetic system, and the body reacts with a primitive physical reaction. Among the effects of this emergency response, the muscles of the shoulder girdle and thoracic spine tense up ready for the impending battle or flight. This further aggravates the malfunction of the sympathetic nerve centres. Under these conditions, the person often feels even more tensed up and a vicious circle is set up.

Inability to cope with a change in routine is another common symptom.

> George, 34, came to me because he was feeling unwell. He had actually missed one appointment already because he couldn't pluck up the courage to come. He had aches in his back, especially in the upper part, as well as mild

85

indigestion. He tired easily and seemed to become tensed up at the slightest thing.

He said that he had missed his earlier appointment because he had great difficulty in doing anything unusual. He was always cancelling dates to go out with friends, and he was finding that he had lost a number of them due to his unreliability.

On examination, he stood with a very curved spine in the thoracic and lumbar regions. His neck movements were about half of normal, and I could feel an intense spasm of the spinal muscles from the skull right down to the sacrum at the bottom of the spine. After 14 treatments to his back, George was 60 per cent better. He found it easier to go out and was markedly more relaxed. When he came back for an assessment after three months, he was 80 per cent improved and only needed two more treatments before he was fully recovered.

Patients such as George find it hard to cope with events out of their normal range of life. This is because the subconscious brain, realizing that the primitive defence mechanism is not working properly, tries to stop them going out of the 'cave'. It suspects that, if they were to meet a wild animal, they might not – without the benefit of a sympathetic nerve boost – be able to cope. Even an invitation to be sociable with friends can seem too daunting, and all sorts of excuses are conjured up in an attempt to avoid something that appears to the subconscious to be confrontational.

In reality, the best possible thing for these people would be to go to the social event. As soon as they arrived, their subconscious would see that there was no danger and they would then be able to enjoy themselves.

THORACIC AND LOWER NECK TROUBLE

We have already seen how trouble in the thoracic and lower neck areas of the spine can depress the activity of the sympathetic nerve ganglia, which lie close to the affected muscles. It follows then that one symptom of HST may be pain in these parts. Patients often complain of fibrositis (inflammation of the fibrous tissue of the muscle sheaths) or non-arthritic pain between the shoulders and/or base of the neck. On examination, there is usually considerable spasm of the paravertebral muscles in the area.

Malfunction of Stellate Ganglion

The disease of HST involves the whole sympathetic system. However, it is more common for only one or two nerve centres to be affected by the build-up of oedema. The particular nerve centre affected will dictate the symptoms. In the context of coronary attacks, we are looking at the stellate ganglion at the base of the neck. It is this group of ganglia which, among other functions, controls the amount of blood passing through the arteries to the brain and to the heart. A malfunction of the stellate ganglion may upset the supply of blood to the heart – but if it does, it does not do so immediately. Indeed, it will be subject to malfunction for some time before the coronary arteries are affected. This may be due to two reasons:

• First, your stellate ganglion controls various parts of your body and so a malfunction may give rise to a number of different ailments. A disruption may, for example, cause a spasm of the arteries to the brain, causing a migraine, or it may affect the arteries to the hands, leading to Reynaud's disease. Or it could affect the supply of blood through the coronary arteries to the heart. This difference in ailments could be partly genetic because of a hereditary difference in the sensitivity of the ganglion in its control of various parts of the body, or it may be due to the fact that the weakest link is the part most easily affected.

- The second reason for the heart being one of the last systems to be affected can be explained by the fact that the body has developed over millions of years and the heart is one of its most primitive parts. As such, it is extremely tough and hard to upset. The more primitive an organ is, the less likely it is to be affected if the sophisticated controls in the body go wrong. There has to be a major disturbance of the sympathetic drive before the heart can be affected.

To explain this second reason more easily, let us look at the effects of alcohol on the layers of the brain. The brain has also developed over the millenia, starting with basic centres which controlled primitive functions, to which have been added over time more and more sophisticated centres. The primitive centres are the toughest and least easily upset by any outside influence such as alcohol. As each layer developed, so they were less tough and more easily disrupted. Then developed consciousness, thinking and, finally, the most delicate of all: the inhibitory centre.

As you drink alcohol, the layers of the brain are affected one by one, and it is the latest-developed and most intricate cells of the inhibitory centre that are affected first. Thus a glass of wine or beer will first make you 'lose your inhibitions' and act in an uncharacteristic way – e.g. a usually shy person may lead the dancing or the resident 'jester' may become gloomy. As you drink more alcohol, the next layer – your thinking centres – are progressively knocked out, so that your thinking becomes less clear and eventually you pass out. Even when you are deeply unconscious, the control over your breathing and the pumping of your heart continues. This is because these functions are the most primitive and thus the hardest to upset. In the same way, the heart is one of the last organs controlled by the stellate ganglion to be affected by any disruption. It is vitally important that this point is fully understood to prevent false alarms – a twinge in the base of the neck does not mean that you are about to have a heart attack!

Reaching Crisis Point

As the congestion around the stellate ganglion increases, the situation will become worse. The cumulative effects of the poor circulation in the area eventually reach such a critical point that the stellate ganglion suddenly withdraws its support almost completely. As the sympathetic pull on a coronary artery lessens, so the parasympathetic system reacts by contracting the muscles of the artery wall and eventually causing it to go into spasm, resulting in a partial or complete blockage of the blood supply to the heart muscle.

This critical point takes several hours, even days, to reach from the first major drop in the sympathetic drive. However, those affected will almost certainly have been suffering from the symptoms of low sympathetic drive.

Alice, aged 57, was a moderately well-known actress. She had been feeling off-colour for two days and, on the third, felt bad enough to see her doctor. She had seen him already some months previously because her indigestion had become somewhat worse, but this had rapidly cleared with medication. The doctor now decided that she was run down and advised her to take at least a day off. Unfortunately, the demanding producer she was working for was not satisfied that she was actually ill, so it was decided that 'the show must go on'.

In the middle of the second act, she suddenly felt dizzy and fainted; her place was taken by her understudy. It was found that she had had a minor coronary thrombosis, and she was off work for several months.

This is a very common story. People very often feel tired or unwell for anything from one to three days before a coronary attack. The crisis can be brought about by a number of factors:

- **Anxiety and worry** over such things as business difficulties can make you tighten all your muscles as if ready for a fight, especially those in the neck and shoulder area, thus diminishing the muscle pump and increasing the local congestion. This is what happened to Alice when she went on stage.
- **Complete rest** also diminishes the workings of the muscle pump. If the activity of the pumping mechanism is already poor due to muscle spasm, a period of rest could reduce it almost to a standstill. Then the congestion in the area becomes too great for the stellate ganglion to cope with. It is for this reason that many people suffer coronary attacks in the early hours of the morning after several hours of complete rest.
- **Unaccustomed exercise.** By the time people reach their 40s, they may be taking little regular exercise,

and the muscles around the stellate ganglion have fewer demands for oxygen. Circulation is maintained at a low, but adequate, level. But as soon as that person gets involved in vigorous exercise, such as a game of squash or a hard run, the muscles need more oxygen, so the blood circulating locally rapidly increases. If there is spasm of the muscles present, the congestion gets worse until there will come a point when, due to lack of oxygen and the build-up of waste products, the stellate ganglion will malfunction, causing a sudden coronary spasm.

• **Weather** can have an adverse affect if you are nearing a coronary attack. The particles in the air – dust, pollens, bacteria, moulds and so on – are ionized. That is, the atoms of which they consist have either gained an extra electron or have lost one, making them either positively or negatively charged. Sunshine and certain terrains such as mountains and the sea tend to make the air more negatively charged. The general level of ionization in the air varies considerably from one day to another.

Wind, wet and darkness tend to make the air more positively charged. Turbulence, including fan heaters, car heating systems and air conditioning, can make the air strongly positive. We also breathe out positively charged particles.

These particles, when inhaled, pass through the walls of the lungs and go into the blood. The negatively charged ones cause no reaction, but the positive ions (atoms or groups of atoms that have gained an electron) react with the platelets in the blood, causing the liberation of one of the brain's chemical transmitters – serotonin. Some of its effects are to make us feel heavy, headachy, lacking in concentration and

91

with diminished judgement, and possibly causing us to be a little bad tempered and aggressive. Most of us recognize the feeling, which is especially common just before a thunderstorm.

Unfortunately, this is not positive ionization's only effect – it also causes the whole body to become congested, with the result that more fluid than normal diffuses into the tissues. This makes any area already congested become even more so, so that symptoms may appear if there were none before, or existing ones may be made worse. This is why the 'prophet' with a touch of 'rheumatics' is able to predict impending rain with some accuracy; the degree of ionization usually changes at least 24 hours before the rain comes.

Positive ionization almost certainly accounts for 'sick building syndrome', when people working in a particular building find the conditions so unpleasant that they feel unwell and cannot work to their full potential. Space saving may result in smaller ventilation ducts; as a consequence, higher-speed air flows increase air turbulence and so the positive ionization.

I have noticed that, on some days as I drive into work in the morning, everyone drives carefully and considerately – 'After you, Fred' and 'Thank you' are the order of the day. A day or so later and everyone is very bad tempered and hot-headed. This gives me a good indication of how my patients will be on that particular day. On the good days, I can be assured that they will mostly be feeling somewhat better.

- **Smoking** paralyses the autonomic nerve centres and this makes arteries contract. One puff of smoke and an artery can remain contracted for some minutes.

Early Diagnosis

There are certain symptoms that become very marked in the few days before the congestion in the area of the stellate ganglion reaches crisis point. There is a very clear clinical picture which you may recognize if you have already suffered a coronary attack, or someone close to you has. This picture builds up over the preceding hours and is identified by *extreme tiredness* and a *tensed-up state*, with perhaps *acute indigestion* and *dizziness on suddenly getting up*.

Severity of the Spasm

The spasm may cause a partial blockage of the coronary artery or a complete close-down, followed by a clot which would make the blockage semi-permanent and may be fatal. This is influenced by several factors:

- **The degree and activity of the disease in the artery.** If the artery is already narrowed by disease, a contraction which was intended, for example, to close the artery down to three-quarters of its diameter may cause a total shutdown. Furthermore, if the disease is recent and active, platelets will stick more readily to the artery walls and there is a higher risk of a clot forming.
- **The amount that the spasm narrows the artery.** If there is only a minor contraction, there may not be enough stagnant blood to form a clot. The degree of spasm directly corresponds to the degree of malfunction of the stellate ganglion. This, in turn, is influenced by the amount of waterlogging in the area of

the neck and thoracic (chest) spine, which is affected
by the severity of the injury to the back and by
conditions such as weather.

- **The duration of the spasm.** If the artery can relax
quickly enough, it may well dilate before any or only
a small clot is formed. This would be particularly so
if there were no disease present in the arterial wall.
If the spasm lasts longer, a major clot may form,
and this will be followed by a full-blown coronary
thrombosis.

5
CORONARY QUESTIONS

There are several anomalies surrounding heart disease which are not easily explained by present-day knowledge, but to which the previous chapter holds the key. This chapter examines these puzzling questions in detail and shows that, to find the answers, one must look beyond the popular theory of arterial disease as the cause of coronary attacks.

Why do people so often feel unwell for up to three days before a heart attack?

If a sudden clot in the artery is the cause of the attack, how can you account for this preliminary period of illness? During the 12–24 hours preceding a heart attack, many people go to their doctors complaining of feeling very unwell and that they are unusually tired and tensed up. They are generally advised to stop work and take things easy.

> Anthony, who was 63 and still very active, had suffered from aches between his shoulders on and off for about 12 years. On Tuesday morning, he was feeling very off colour and tired. Indeed, he felt so unwell, he went to see his GP, who examined him but found nothing abnormal. The doctor told Antony to take it easy for a day or so.
>
> That evening, Anthony felt so much better that he went

to see some friends. But as the evening went on, he started to have bad attacks of indigestion and then a pain in his left shoulder and arm. He suddenly collapsed unconscious, and his friends called an ambulance. When he arrived at hospital, it was found that he had suffered a coronary attack and he was taken to intensive care. Thankfully, he survived.

It is my belief that, when someone like Anthony feels so unwell, the possibility that this might be a precursor to a heart attack should always be considered. The person may be suffering from a sudden sharp drop in the sympathetic drive, which is about to reach the critical point, giving rise to a spasm of a coronary artery.

Why is it that when people, who have just suffered massive heart attacks, arrive at hospital, the tests – even an ECG – can be completely normal?

If a clot had caused the coronary blockage, it would still be present, shutting off the blood supply to a part of the heart muscle; in this case, the local damage to the heart would be considerable. The ECG would detect the effect of the clot on the pumping action of the muscle, and the blood tests that detect any products of the breaking up of muscles would be abnormal. When a muscle is damaged, some of it dies and proteins are released as it disintegrates. The level of these breakdown products can be measured to assess the degree of damage to the heart muscle.

Peter, a 49-year-old solicitor, was sitting at his desk when he suffered a bad attack of pain on the left side of his chest and down his left arm. He went straight to hospital, but his ECG and blood tests were all normal. However,

the pain had been so severe that he was put on a cor.
regime.

The trouble soon subsided, but five months later, he felt
the pains again and he went back to hospital. He also
had the same outcome: no signs of abnormality in his ECG
or his blood tests.

On his third attack, he came to me and I found that he
had tremendous spasm of the upper thoracic paravertebral
muscles and a very tender second thoracic vertebra. After
six sessions of treatment with my form of physical medicine, Peter said he had not felt so well in a very long time.
Six years later, the pains have still not recurred.

Why did all of Peter's tests show normal results? The
answer is that the blockage was caused by a spasm of the
coronary artery which had subsided by the time he reached
hospital. In such a case as Peter's, there was too little
disease in the artery to make it vulnerable to a thrombosis,
so the muscle remained completely undamaged.

*Most arteries in the body are prone to disease, so why
is it usually only the coronary and cerebral arteries
that cause any trouble?*

If disease alone causes blockages in arteries, many of our
arte. es would be as vulnerable to a thrombosis as the
coronary arteries. Other factors must be involved.

As I have already explained, the coronary and cerebral
arteries differ from other arteries in that their role requires
them to change their internal diameters rapidly and with
amazing precision from being very dilated to being very
small. If other arteries are diseased, there is usually still
plenty of room for blood to pass through, even in their
most contracted state. However, with a coronary artery, it

takes only a small amount of disease and then a spasm to close it off completely, thus running the risk of a clot.

> Sarah, a 57-year-old designer, considered herself to be of average fitness, although she took little exercise. One morning at breakfast, she suddenly felt ill with a severe pain in her chest and numbness in her left shoulder, which radiated a little into her left arm. She was brought into hospital but died the next day.
>
> The post-mortem examination showed a thrombosis in one of her coronary arteries. There was atherosclerosis at the site of the thrombosis, but this was slight and almost certainly not enough in itself to have caused the clot.

It is known that arterial disease comes on slowly and remains relatively constant. Yet people often recover from one attack and lead perfectly normal lives only to suffer another attack several months later. If there is enough disease to cause a thrombosis on one day, how do you account for the periods between attacks when the level of disease remains unchanged?

The answer is that a blockage of the artery is not caused solely by disease but is the result of a spasm of a diseased artery. The story of one of my patients who subsequently became a great friend illustrates this anomaly.

> Mike, a 58-year-old stockbroker, had 14 heart attacks in the space of only three years. Soon after his third attack, he was advised to retire as it was likely that he would suffer another in the near future. Mike ignored this advice. He came to me after his 14th attack, saying he was at his wit's end. He didn't want to give up work but he was seriously worried about his health – why did the attacks keep recurring?

During his first visit, I felt a spasm from the back of his skull to the vertebrae in his lower back. He also revealed that he became tired very easily and always seemed to feel tensed up. He had fibrositis between his shoulders and had suffered from indigestion for about 15 years.

Mike had such a low sympathetic drive that it was causing spasms of the coronary artery. I gave him treatment over three months, with 14 visits in all. He felt so well afterwards that he continued with his job, dying of pneumonia 21 years later, aged 79, having had no further heart problems.

Many heart attacks occur in the early hours of the morning. If the level of disease is constant day and night, how can this be explained?

Simon, 42, was a large man who had been out of work for several years. He was very tense about financial problems and tried to relax by taking a lot of exercise. He had bouts of indigestion and got tired very easily, symptoms which he put down to his difficult circumstances.

Then one night at about 2.45 a.m, he awoke with a bad attack of indigestion. He tried taking antacids but the pain in his stomach became worse, and after about three quarters of an hour, he sent for a doctor. His pulse was weak and his blood pressure low. On reaching hospital, an ECG confirmed that he had had a coronary thrombosis. He was in hospital for three weeks.

Many people like Simon have heart attacks in bed during the night. Why? To answer that, we need to take another look at the pumping mechanism in the muscles, which circulates blood back to the heart. This mechanism is activated by movement of the muscles; during rest, the action is minimal. In a healthy body at rest, an adequate circulation is maintained by a combination of the residual pressure from the heart, waves of contractions up the vein walls ('milking' the blood up the vessel) and the minimal movements that a person makes when asleep. However, if the person already has a spasm of the muscles of the back, causing oedema in the tissues, prolonged rest can cause a sufficient increase in the tissue fluid to result in a crisis of the sympathetic nerve system. In such circumstances, this would give rise to a spasm of the coronary artery.

Why does a post-mortem sometimes show that a myocardial infarct (death of part of the heart muscle resulting from the blockage of the blood supply) precedes a coronary thrombosis?

There have been several occasions when pathologists have found that a thrombosis actually formed after a patient died, so it was clearly not the cause of death. This happened to Freda, the 51-year-old mother of three teenagers. Much to the great distress of her family, Freda died suddenly at home. When her body was examined at post-mortem, a clot (thrombus) was found in one of the coronary arteries. However, this was deemed to have come about after her death when the stationary blood reacted with some roughening of the artery wall. This obviously meant that the clot could not have caused the fatal attack. So what was the cause? The answer was that Freda had such a depleted sympathetic drive that it caused the coronary artery to go into spasm. As the artery was already narrowed by disease, this spasm was enough to close off the blood supply to the heart muscle, causing an infarct. The formation of the clot occurred as a natural sequence of events after Freda died. The fatal stoppage of blood was caused by the spasm, not the thrombosis.

Why do some cardiac patients have histories of transient dizzy spells for several years before their heart attacks?

Harry, a 49-year-old postman, had a mild heart attack and was brought to hospital. He told me that he had been seeing doctors for about 12 years because he had dizzy spells. These spells, which lasted for several minutes, came on at different times of the day and didn't seem to be brought on by anything special. Investigations had not shown any particular cause. However, an ECG revealed signs of previous slight damage to the heart muscle, and the dizzy spells were thought to have been very minor heart attacks.

My view of Harry's medical history is that he had been suffering from low sympathetic drive. This had caused a number of minor spasms of one of his coronary arteries, which had been enough to make his heart falter and cause the dizzy spells, but not enough to give rise to any serious problem. Then his sympathetic drive had finally dropped enough, or the spasm had lasted long enough, to cause a minor heart attack.

It cannot be emphasized too strongly that there are, of course, many other much more common causes of dizziness, but if none of these is diagnosed, then, with patients such as Harry, the possibility of low sympathetic drive should be considered.

Why should a relatively fit person suffer a heart attack while playing squash or jogging?

David, 47, was an active gardener who played regular games of football and squash. He liked to lead life to the full, although he did have indigestion and tired very easily once he got home after a day's work.

He was playing squash one night at about 8 p.m. when

he remarked that he had a cramp-like pain in his chest and then suddenly collapsed. On arriving at hospital, a coronary thrombosis was diagnosed, and after a spell in the intensive care unit, he made a good recovery.

If you watch a squash player (like David) or a jogger in action, you will see that the muscles in the neck have to work very hard to hold the head in a stationary position on top of the moving body. Although the muscles are working extra hard, there may not be sufficient movement of them to activate the muscle pump to return into the veins the greatly increased blood flow they require. This is especially true if there is a great deal of tension involved, as this causes a considerable tightening of the shoulder muscles. This will result in greater congestion of the neck area and will eventually disrupt the stellate ganglion to such an extent that a coronary spasm results.

Statistics show that the peak age for heart attacks is between 40 and 55. How can you account for this?

The muscles of men (who are much more prone to heart attacks than women) are still very strong at this age. In addition, many of them have injured their backs in the past, often without realizing it. This is also an age when people become less involved in exercise yet still consider themselves fairly active. They are likely to place a lot of intermittent and unaccustomed demands on their bodies, doing tasks such as chopping wood or moving heavy furniture.

The congestion in the neck area from an old injury would be considerably increased by such activity: the muscles are still powerful, and the increase in the blood supply to meet their needs when exercising can all too easily flood the area. The combination of unaccustomed exercise with a diseased artery makes such a person vulnerable to a coronary episode.

By the age of 65 or so, all the muscles in the body become weaker. It follows that the protective spasm across the facet joints could be correspondingly weaker, and in my experience, there is often a spontaneous improvement in the back's condition. This leads to an easing of the congestion around the stellate ganglion and reduces the risk of a coronary attack.

The incidence of coronary attacks used to be far higher in men than in women, but the pendulum is starting to swing back. Why is this so?

Although men are still at the greatest risk of a coronary attack, more and more women are becoming vulnerable. This is because, until some decades ago, women were far less likely to participate in strenuous activities, so their muscles were correspondingly weaker. As a result, the spasm across the facet joints was less intense and the congestion of the back and associated tissues was less severe than in men. Now that women are taking part in a wider range of competitive sports, they are suffering more injuries and also developing stronger muscles. In these circumstances, one would expect a closing of the gap between the incidence of coronary attacks in the two sexes. The protection of the arteries in women is another reason why I so strongly advocate the use of hormone replacement therapy when needed (*See* page 46).

A number of factors are known to increase the risk of a coronary attack. Yet despite the variety and number of these factors, no less than two thirds of all people who have attacks have no known risk factor. Why is this?

To counter this puzzling fact, I would like to reveal another interesting statistic. The number of people who have trouble with their backs at chest level (i.e. the thoracic spine) is almost identical to the number of people suffering coronary attacks – i.e. about 40 per cent. This statistic, which backs up my theory, should not be ignored. When you are dealing with such large numbers of people vulnerable to a serious illness, it is imperative that all avenues be explored in the prevention of attacks.

Management of a Coronary Problem

The next chapter looks at the different factors involved in the management of a coronary problem. Briefly, these can be divided into three parts:

1 The detection of the vulnerability of a person to a possible heart attack, and then treatment to minimize the risk of the attack actually occurring.
2 The management of the patient at the time of the actual attack, followed by the skilled follow-up, preferably in a specialized cardiac hospital unit.
3 Preventative treatment that is given once the patient has fully recovered from an attack, to avoid a further attack.

The care that needs to be given immediately following a coronary episode is outside the scope of this book, other than to emphasize the importance of calling for skilled

104

medical help and learning the resuscitation techniques that could keep a person alive until either this help arrives or the heart resumes an adequate beat. The first and third management aspects are central to my treatment. It is the ability to form a long-term view that a risk may be present, and then, even more importantly, the ability to give a reasonably effective treatment for prevention of the attack that are the unique features of this book.

6

MENDING A BROKEN HEART

As I was sitting down to write the introduction to this chapter, a postcard arrived on my desk from one of my patients on holiday in Norway. 'Never felt better,' she wrote.

Twelve months previously, Julie, a 27-year-old air hostess, had come to me with symptoms of low sympathetic drive: excessive tiredness, indigestion, headaches, bouts of mild depression, and fibrositis between her shoulder blades. She had also had a few mild fainting attacks that had lasted several minutes. Julie had been working long hours and didn't think she could cope much longer. Her doctor had been able to offer little positive help.

After a thorough examination, I diagnosed symptoms of low sympathetic drive. I explained that, if the underlying condition was not treated, there was a slight risk of a more serious complication. She agreed to treatment, and within several months, her condition and quality of life had improved dramatically. If Julie's condition had not been diagnosed, she may have been at risk of a heart attack. By treating the fundamental cause, I was able greatly to eliminate this risk (if it had indeed been present) and also improve her general health beyond measure.

On a less happy note, there have been three occasions

when I have seen patients for a small problem and, after listening to their medical histories and examining them, have decided that they were at some risk of a coronary attack. In each case, for differing reasons, they were unable or unwilling to undergo treatment, and each had a coronary thrombosis within the following 18 months.

One was the 64-year-old wife of a neighbour, whom I saw one evening as she had a very painful back; she regarded me simply as 'the gardener next door' and saw little reason to follow my advice. The second was a shop keeper whose establishment I visited often. He came to me for a consultation because of intermittent back trouble. Despite my warning, he said he was a busy man and he felt that it would have to be a major problem before he would come for treatment.

The third patient was a senior adminstrator of the Royal Homoeopathic Hospital, who consulted me about his painful toe. I examined him and, among other things, found that he had a great deal of oedema at the base of his neck, muscle spasm in this area and a history of several dizzy spells and one momentary blackout over the past few years. I explained that his toe was a relatively easy problem, but he had another trouble that could cause anxiety in a year or two, so he should have treatment as soon as possible to rectify this as well. He said that he was about to make his annual three-month visit to Barbados, and that as soon as he got back, he would take my advice and have treatment. Unfortunately, he never returned to England: just over two months later, he had a massive coronary attack and died in Barbados.

Thankfully, I cannot remember any other patients whom I saw and felt that they were nearing a critical phase but who refused treatment.

Broadly speaking, my patients can be divided into three

groups: those such as Julie who have the obvious symptoms and signs of low sympathetic drive and who would like to feel better in their general health; those who are experiencing anginal pain; and those who have already had a heart attack and, having got over it, would like to minimize the residual effects and also take steps to reduce the probability of a further attack. This chapter will show how, through correct diagnosis and treatment, such people can be helped. I believe it is possible greatly to reduce the risks of getting a first attack and also, equally importantly, to avoid another attack in those who have already had one.

A CAUTIONARY NOTE

Before continuing, I would like to stress that my treatment is not a substitute for conventional, orthodox medicine. The advice and treatment given by cardiologists is of the very highest standard. The knowledge that the medical profession has concerning both prevention and treatment is one of the miracles of modern times. However, it is my hope that this book will add an extra dimension to the treatment of coronary attacks.

Beta-Blockers – the Anomoly

It is worth considering one aspect of the drug treatment of coronary trouble. Beta-blockers are commonly used as they damp down the whole sympathetic–adrenalin mechanism. Beta-receptors are the adrenalin activity-producing part of the sympathetic nervous system. By blocking them, the activity of the sympathetic nervous system is reduced in proportion to the amount of drug given. There is, however, an anomaly in the use of beta-blockers: if low sympathetic drive causes a coronary attack, a drug to lower the sympathetic drive further would hardly seem appropriate as a treatment for the attack.

However, by lowering the whole activity of the body, including the output of the heart muscle, beta-blockers ensure that the heart has a great deal less work to do, and while its blood supply is impeded, as it would be due to arterial disease or spasm, this is the all-important consideration. Beta-blockers also lower blood pressure, further assisting the heart by cutting its load. There are a number of beta-blocker drugs, and they all have slightly different effects on the person taking them as they work on different parts of the sympathetic nervous system. In addition, the effects of the same drug can be different in different people.

If the stellate ganglia is the centre of the cause of the coronary thrombosis, this is because it is in an area of oedema where the tissue circulation is very poor. For this reason, any drug given by mouth will have little, if any, effect on it. This means that the rest of the body will benefit from the beta-blocker without a major adverse effect on the size of the coronary arteries themselves – i.e. the drug will not decrease the internal diameters of these arteries. So oedema around the stellate ganglion may explain the anomaly of why a drug that is supposed to reduce the diameters of the coronary arteries can actually be of use in the treatment of heart trouble.

Using Physical Medicine (Treatment using massage, manipulation and electrical and other equipment)

My treatment relies on physical medicine which has the great advantage that, provided all reasonable precautions are taken, it involves almost no risk and has no side-effects. One of my favourite sayings is: 'The risk of any treatment that you give to a patient must never exceed the risk of not giving the treatment.' As hyposympathetic tone (HST) poses no obvious or immediate threat to patients' lives, it would not be justified to administer any risky treatment to relieve it. Clearly, if a patient has actually had a coronary attack, some risk might be permissible in an attempt to avoid another one. Fortunately, however, no risk is actually involved with this physical treatment.

The lynchpins of my treatment are surged faradism (an electric pulse that causes the muscles to contract, thus activating the muscle pump), massage, remobilization and manipulation, and ultrasonic waves. Many patients who come to me with back pain have been to a variety of different practitioners who have used these treatments. Since they did little to relieve symptoms then, they ask me, why should they help now? In answer, I stress that it is necessary to distinguish between the tools used to carry out the treatment and the treatment itself.

To illustrate this, consider a piece of land that is not producing good crops. No one has any idea why the soil has turned foul. Land experts are called in, and they try to improve conditions by digging up the land or weeding and fertilizing it using spades, forks and hoes. It is all to no avail – the land is still not fruitful. Then another expert comes along and suggests that the problem may be that the ditches around the plot are blocked resulting in poor drainage. He uses the same spades, forks and hoes to clear the ditches. This time it works. His success lies not in the types of tools he used but in the way he viewed the problem. He used the same tools as the others but achieved quite different results through a totally different approach to the problem.

Treating the Basic Problem

To undertand how my treatment works, it is necessary to recapitulate. A heart attack is preceded by a past injury such as a fall down stairs, a slip on a hard floor or a car accident which gave a jolt to your spine. This blow bruises the tiny facet joints between the affected vertebrae in your back. As a result of the bruising, the muscles across these facet joints go into a powerful contraction called a spasm.

There is a mechanism in the body whereby impulses, originating in bruised joints, travel along nerves to the spinal cord and then go straight to the muscles across the joint, putting them into spasm (*see* Fig. 4.6, p. 75). This produces an effect rather like a corset of muscles which is designed to limit movement, thereby giving the joints a rest and speeding their recovery. Unfortunately the repair mechanism of the back does not work as intended. The spasm puts tremendous pressure on the facet joints and does very little to limit movement. The joints are not rested, and every time they move, the strain is greatly increased.

This unfortunate situation is further aggravated by the fact that an important function of the muscles is to return blood to the heart from the tissues. Every time a muscle contracts, the tissues tighten both in the muscle and in adjacent areas. This forces fluid out of the tissue spaces into the veins where non-return valves ensure that it makes steady progress back to the heart. As the muscles in a spasm are permanently contracted, this pumping effect is interfered with and leads to excessive fluid, known as oedema, collecting in the area (*see* Fig. 4.7b, p. 79). The build-up of oedema has the effect of diminishing the circulation to the tissues, which not only delays recovery of the damage to the joints but results in further deterioration.

The traffic jam gets worse and spreads to nearby tissues, causing congestion and disruption of their normal functioning. In the context of this book, the most important of the tissues to be affected are those that comprise the sympathetic nervous system, whose uppermost group of nerve centres, the stellate ganglion, lies at the base of the neck. A malfunction of the sympathetic nervous system will eventually give rise to the symptoms of HST, a new disease that was described in detail in Chapter 4. After some length of time, if the congestion is very bad, it may disturb one of the most basic functions of the stellate ganglion – the control of the narrowing and dilation of the coronary arteries. The malfunction of the stellate ganglion, combined with disease of the arterial wall, contracts the internal diameters of the coronary arteries (*see* Fig. 1.11a & b, p. 31 and Fig. 3.2a & b, p. 56) and obstructs the flow of blood to the heart. This could finally lead to a heart attack.

EASING THE CONGESTION

Clearly, the stellate ganglion must be 'dried out' if the risks of a heart attack are to be reduced. However, to do so, the fundamental problem must be addressed – that is, the bruised facet joints which have caused the powerful protective spasm of the muscles in the neck and upper thoracic (chest) area. The object of my treatment is to promote suitable local conditions for the body to heal these damaged joints.

The treatment has three basic aims:

- To reduce the muscle spasm as much as possible to take some of the pressure off the joints.
- To improve the tissue circulation around the facet joints by squeezing out the stagnant oedema in the tissue spaces and making room for fresh fluid to filter in.
- To stretch the muscles and ligaments across the damaged vertebrae that have shortened during the prolonged muscle spasm. These tend to shorten to take up the slack when the muscle is in spasm, thus compressing the vertebrae together for a long time. Unless they are made to revert to their former length, they will continue to exert pressure on the joint surfaces and so interfere with a full recovery, even when the muscles have relaxed their spasm and thus eliminated this pressure on the joints.

Tools of the Treatment

My treatment relies on a number of different 'tools':

Surged fardism, in the form of a 'square wave pulse', is applied to the nerves which supply the muscles in the neck and thoracic area. This is probably one of the most important parts of the treatment. It acts to make the muscles contract and relax in a rhythmical way at the optimum speed, thus forcing the muscle pump to work. Once the muscles start pumping the oedema out of the area, the congestion is eased – not only in the immediate locality but also in nearby areas including that of the sympathetic nervous system.

Interferential treatment (another form of electrical treatment) is often substituted by physiotherapists. However, since this does not activate the muscle pump in the same way as surged faradism, it is not nearly as effective. Patients who have been given interferential treatment rarely make proper progress.

The success of faradism depends on precise timing and strength. It must not be given at too strong a level or for too long a time as the extra muscular activity would greatly increase the arterial blood supply. As the increased supply would continue for some while following treatment, it would flood the area again, interfering with the tissue circulation and upsetting the treatment. Around three minutes on each muscle group seems to be a good average time for faradism.

Massage of the affected muscles. Firm but gentle massage encourages the muscle to come out of spasm. It also helps to squeeze the oedema out of the surrounding area into the veins, thus relieving some of the congestion. As with faradism, the intensity and duration of the massage must be correct to achieve maximum benefit. It must be firm enough to produce the desired effects, but not so vigorous or prolonged as to stimulate and increase the arterial supply so that it will flood the area later.

Remobilization and manipulation of the thoracic spine plays a vital role by attempting to ensure reasonably permanent protection. When a spinal muscle is in spasm, the vertebrae are pulled together, thus compressing the elastic intervertebral discs. After a time, the ligaments and muscle

114

fibres contract to take up the slack. So, even when the muscle spasm is relaxed, there is little improvement as the shortened structures continue to exert considerable pressure on the facet joints. Repeated, forced remobiliz-ation or manipulation can stretch them back to the right length and help keep the muscle from going back into spasm.

Ultrasonic waves are the least important of my treatment tools. These are sound waves that hit a far higher note than a human or even a dog can hear. If you have good hearing, you can hear around 17,000 vibrations a second; the frequency used in my practice is 3,000,000 vibrations a second (3 MHz). Recently we have been using a new type of machine with a frequency of 680 KHz and this seems even more effective.

When ultrasonic waves at a strength above about 2 watts to the square centimetre (a very weak dose) are applied to muscles in spasm, they have the effect of con-tracting the arterioles somewhat, which lessens the exces-sive supply of blood to the area and helps to ease the traffic jam. On average, I use about 2 watts to the square centimetre, which is effective and yet low enough to be comfortable for the patient.

Ultrasonic waves also speed up chemical reactions, probably by buffeting molecules about so they meet other ones more frequently. This, of course, makes the healing process much faster. They are also thought to alter the filtration pressure of the tissue fluid by making some of the big protein molecules stick together, thereby increas-ing the osmotic, or filtration, pressure in the tissue fluid. This causes the fluid to be drawn out of the area, back into the blood vessels.

Lastly, ultrasonic waves also encourage muscles to come

out of a cramp or spasm. If the waves are applied directly over the facet joints, this also greatly speeds up the repair processes in them. Patients will almost always improve without the use of ultrasonic waves, but the recovery will take longer.

OTHER TOOLS

Application of cold is used if the person has a great deal of pain at the base of the neck or upper chest region – in the form of a cold spray or pack of frozen peas, preferably petit pois! When applied to the neck and thoracic area, the cold will chill the locality. This must only be used for up to about ½ minute, just long enough to chill the area down thoroughly. The body reacts to the cooling effect by closing down the arterial circulation in an attempt to conserve heat by limiting the amount of blood becoming chilled. This means that less fluid diffuses *into* the tissue spaces, and so it follows that less fluid has to diffuse *out* to maintain equilibrium.

In fact, the drainage will usually exceed the flow in for a while, which has a number of beneficial effects. The change in the ratio of big-flow-in and small-flow-out to smaller-flow-in and bigger-flow-out is seen at its most obvious when there is a bad swelling, such as in a sprained ankle. The application of cold reduces the swelling rapidly and helps greatly to accelerate recovery. A somewhat less obvious example of this can be seen when someone receives a blow in the face: the application of ice or frozen peas will limit the eventual bruising very considerably. The traditional steak for a black eye probably worked partly because it was cold and partly because the pressure caused by holding the steak to the eye compressed the tissues and prevented blood flowing into them.

Arteries are like reinforced hosepipes with fluid under high pressure running through them. Even if you tread on such a pipe, you would not be able to compress it to lessen the flow. Veins, on the other hand, are like thin plastic tubes with little pressure in the fluid flowing through them. The trouble with this state of affairs is that, if the surrounding pressure goes up somewhat, it can readily compress veins, obstructing their ability to drain an area, but the increase in pressure will have very little effect on diminishing the flow through arteries. This results in even more fluid collecting in the tissues and, as can be seen in the case of the sprained ankle, a large swelling can develop.

The situation in the back is similar, although the build-up of oedema would not be nearly as bad as with the ankle. However, it can be seen that, if the veins and lymphatic ducts are compressed, even to a small extent, this will reduce the tissue circulation somewhat. If cold lowers the pressure in the tissue fluids, it can actually *increase* the tissue circulation, so it is a positive measure assisting recovery. Heat, of course, increases arterial flow and drives fluid into the area, giving a feeling of comfort as oxygen is taken into the deprived area. But it then compresses the drainage, bringing the tissue circulation to a standstill.

A further advantage of cold is that it also slows down the tissues' metabolism – the speed of all the chemical reactions – so that the requirements of oxygen are correspondingly less.

Cold also reduces the sensitivity of the nerves. We all feel that it is harder to move around when we are cold. This means that the impulses that would have been transmitted to the muscles from the bruised area are greatly diminished, and the protective spasm is therefore reduced proportionately. The reduction of pressure on the facet joints and possible slight improvement in the muscle pump both help speed recovery.

Of course, this major reduction in the conduction of the nerve impulses can also greatly diminish the sensation of pain. The effect can be dramatic, and by the time the nerves have recovered their function, the other effects mentioned may well have produced sufficient improvement to have relieved the pain completely.

Anti-inflammatory drugs may also be used in recommended doses, as they can offer a worthwhile reduction in the time required to obtain a good recovery. These drugs neutralize chemical messengers in the body called prostaglandins, which are involved in the production of inflammation.

Aspirin. It has been shown that an aspirin a day by limiting the clotting mechanism of the blood confers some protection against a coronary thrombosis. Is such a little dose really enough to affect the probability of a clot? Well, it seems likely to me that it will damp down the inflammation in the back's facet joints, lessening the spasm and thus reducing the oedema around the stellate ganglion. In fact, this common drug may, like others, have more than one effect.

Exercise. My patients are encouraged to follow a daily five-minute exercise plan (*see* Appendix 1) designed to increase the efficiency of the muscle pump in the back and neck and keep the muscles in good working order. It's also wise to make general exercise part of your everyday routine. Regular exercise helps keep your heart muscles fit and strong, which both reduces your risks of an attack and (if you should be so unfortunate as to have one) increases your chances of making a full recovery afterwards. Violent exercise that is sufficient to make you breathless should be taken at least weekly.

All muscles vary in size and strength according to the amount of work they do – and the heart is no exception. So if a cardiac patient is told to rest, the heart has relatively little work to do. As a result, the muscle will quickly deteriorate and grow smaller and weaker. If, on the other hand, the patient takes up regular exercise, the heart will become stronger and fitter, and the patient is able to cope with the demands of everyday activities and stands a far higher chance of surviving future heart attacks.

As everyone's exercise needs and desires are so different, it is impossible to give a set programme of general exercise. It is up to you (preferably in consultation with your GP or cardiologist) to devise you own individual routine, incorporating a variety of different forms of exercise.

Positive attitude of mind has a great influence on the ability of your body to repair itself. Just as people are split into those who rejoice that their glass is half-full and those who complain that their glass is half-empty, so the attitudes of cardiac patients are divided. Some feel so lucky that they have survived an attack that they resolve to stay fit and live a long time, while others feel that the sword of Damocles is suspended by a hair six inches above their head and spend their life in constant dread of another attack. Unfortunately, the latter is all too often a self-perpetuating philosophy, but it doesn't always have to be that way.

Mary had suffered a mild coronary thrombosis and was in a very depressed frame of mind. She was worried about how she would cope at home and how she would look

119

after her husband on his return from a business trip to Australia. As her spirits sank deeper and deeper, she seemed to lose all incentive to get better. Thankfully, her husband cut his trip short and was home within a few days. It was touching to see how pleased they were to see each other. As Mary's face lit up, it was as if someone had flicked on an electric light. With her husband's encouragement, she adopted a more positive outlook on life and recovered rapidly.

It is important that those who have had heart attacks should live as normal a life as they possibly can, as this is much better for morale. When people come to me for treatment, I often suggest that they let up a little on any rigorous regime prescribed by their consultants. If they have been taken off foods or drinks they enjoy, for example, I advise them to eat or drink them in great moderation. Many patients say they feel much better, even before the 'real' treatment begins, at the mere thought of being able to enjoy a small brandy at the end of the day. A normal lifestyle is also physically better for the patient. If you get out and move about more, you keep the muscle pump active and recovery is speeded up. If you lie around in bed or on the sofa and worry, you are hindering your body's natural repair mechanisms.

Many years ago, a great friend of mine had a severe coronary thrombosis at the age of 62. She was the thin, active type who had enjoyed life in every aspect and who had been very fit until the heart attack struck her down. Imagine, therefore, her dismay when she was told by the foremost heart specialist of the day that, if she wished to see another year, she would have to live the life of a cabbage. She was advised to move her bed to the ground floor of her house to avoid the exertion of stairs, and not to get up until after lunch. She was allowed to potter about in the garden until tea time, after which it would be wise for her to return to bed. The alternative? If she was any more active than this, her prospects for survival may well be only a few weeks.

Following a short conference with her very supportive husband, she decided to go down with all flags flying. A trip to Switzerland was rapidly arranged so that she could fulfil the wish of her lifetime: as a keen gardener, she had always wanted to see the Alpine plants at their best and this was the ideal time of year.

She tramped over the Alps for six weeks and returned with a crate of plants for her own beautiful garden. The following year, she went again, and by the time her heart finally claimed her – after 17 fit and active years – she was reputed to have one of the finest collections of Alpine plants in Britain.

There is a small twist to the story. On the fourth year, she brought back plants for her cardiologist who was also renowned for his garden. When he looked a little annoyed by the present, she said: 'You know, James, you would much rather have sent me flowers to prove that you were correct than to receive them from me which proves that you were wrong in your original advice.'

Support from family and close friends also helps recovery. If patients come to my practice with their husbands or wives, the spouses are invited to join the consultation. This is for two reasons. First, they often remember past injuries and early symptoms far better than the patient: 'You had a bad tumble down the stairs the year after we were married' or 'You complained of a dreadful ache after planting those bulbs four summers ago.' The patient may not feel such information is relevant, but it is most helpful to me.

Second, if the patient's partner and family understands what I am aiming to achieve with the treatment and how it can help prevent future attacks, I can usually rely on them to keep the patient on the straight and narrow. A wife, for example, will remind her husband to do his daily exercises; a husband will ensure that his wife continues coming for treatment until the problem is cleared up. It is so important that families work together to help restore the patient to good health. Sadly, this was not the case with Miles, who always seemed so cheery.

> Miles was in hospital. He had had a minor coronary thrombosis, followed by pneumonia and pleurisy, but fortunately was making a good recovery. He was the life and soul of the ward, and if any patient was a bit miserable, Miles could be relied upon to be there with a friendly word. Any nurse who was a bit pushed could be sure that help was at hand. Miles told us all about his wonderful family and home. He said that, when his 'super' son Martin had married, Miles had bought a big house and let Martin and his new wife live in it. Miles occupied a bed-sitting room, completely self-contained, on the first floor, and said that he enjoyed helping out with the babysitting and shopping.
>
> It seemed sad that none of us knew what Martin, the wonderful son, actually looked like, as, for one reason after another, he had never managed to make the journey to the hospital to visit his father. Never mind, said Miles, it would all be made up in the celebrations when at last he returned home. When Miles was well enough, we got in touch with his son to say that he could pick up his father at the end of the week. 'I don't mind what you do with the old fool', the son said. 'We're sick of his jokes and stupid stories. Find an old peoples' home or something for him – we'll never have him back here.'

Miles went quiet at the news and just sat, silent, in his bed. He never really said anything again. One day kind fate took a hand: Miles did not wake up that morning. He had had a massive coronary thrombosis and slipped away into peaceful oblivion. Had he had something to live for, we were all sure that Miles would have continued to spread his own particular brand of sunshine on all around him for many more years.

Upsetting though this story is, it is important to remember that the opposite of this story must be equally true. Help, support and love go a long way to maximize a patient's own repair mechanism so that he or she will recover more quickly and completely than they would have done without this support.

Your Questions Answered

When should I come for the sort of treatment outlined in this book?

Anyone who is showing obvious signs of a low sympathetic drive should be checked over. The symptoms do not necessarily mean that a heart attack is imminent, but it is sensible to be checked as a precautionary measure. You may recognize the symptoms in yourself or in someone close to you:

- aches between the shoulders or in the neck.
- extreme tiredness which tends to peak at around 3.00 in the afternoon. Sufferers tend to have the energy to cope when under pressure, even an ordinary day's work, but become very tired as soon as they relax.

123

- indigestion, headaches and dizzy spells, and the tendency to get tensed up very easily.

Whether or not these symptoms are indicative of a vulnerability to a heart attack, they deserve treatment in their own right. The majority of my patients say they didn't realize how bad they were feeling before they had treatment; they had thought that, apart from discomfort, they were perfectly well. It is rather like looking around a room and wondering if it needs redecorating. The tendency is to leave it for a year or so. It is only when you have given the room a new coat of paint that you realize how tatty it was before. If your health deteriorates slowly, you won't be aware that it is going downhill because you can't recall what it was like to be normal. It's not until your health is restored that you appreciate just how ill you had been feeling.

> Reggie, aged 54 had had a sudden pain in his chest as he had hurried after a bus five years previously. Fortunately it had gone off quickly as soon as he had sat down in the bus. Relieved, he had forgotten all about it and carried on with his life. Unfortunately, not long afterwards, he had had another attack of pain as he was walking his dog. Worried, he had gone immediately to his doctor, who had sent him to the hospital to be investigated. He had been found to have a slight narrowing of one of his coronary arteries, but it had been judged to be too slight to justify surgery.
>
> He came to see me to discover if anything could be done to minimize his chest pain, which was not only a nuisance but also posed a continual threat to him. Apart from the angina, he tired very easily and had troublesome indigestion and mild fibrositis between his shoulders. I found a great deal of spasm in his paravertebral muscles from the

124

neck to the lumbar region. He had treatment to that part of the spine, at the end of which he felt better than he had for years, lost his indigestion and tensed-up state and, after five years, had not had another pain in his chest.

If you have already had a coronary, you should seek this sort of preventative treatment as soon as you have been released from the immediate care you received following the attack and you have returned to some sort of normality. It is important not to have preventative treatment too soon as it is very tiring. Your body is already working at full stretch to put your heart right, so you don't want to divert energy from this vital task.

Does the treatment hurt?

This is a common concern, but fortunately, the answer is no. Indeed, many patients find it very relaxing and often comment that they know instinctively that it is working. Of course, there may be the occasional twinge, but the principle of the treatment is that it must not hurt. It is important to remember that the treatment is only trying to put the repair mechanism into order so that the body can heal itself. The treatment, on its own, cannot actually repair anything. If it hurts, the body is going to regard it as an enemy and react against it, so blocking any beneficial effect.

How many treatment sessions will I need?

This is a difficult question to answer as there can be so many variations of the basic problem. However, the average seems to be around six to 12 visits. Some patients need fewer sessions, some need many more.

For the treatment to be successful, it is essential to see

it through to the end. It is rather like pushing a sledge up a snowy slope. If you leave it 10 feet from the top and go home for dinner, it will have slipped some distance down the slope by the time you get back. If you push it right to the top before you leave, it is far more likely to stay there.

The measure of a patient's recovery is the degree of spasm in the muscles which can be felt by palpation. The last bits of spasm can be quite difficult to feel, so it is always hard to know exactly when you can tell patients that they have made a full recovery. It is for this reason that I ask patients to return in three months for a further check to see if any more treatment is required.

After the first treatment, there is a marked improvement in the conditions needed for the repair of the facet joints: the muscles are more relaxed; the stale oedema has been pumped out of their tissue spaces and they have refreshed fluid in them. The joints will begin to heal and the spasm will begin to become less intense.

However, after a day or so, when the repair has improved the situation about 10 to 20 per cent, the body mechanism, thinking that it knows best, puts the muscles back into spasm, thus halting the repair. By the time the patient comes back for the second treatment, the spasm is then usually around 10 per cent better. After this and subsequent treatments, the same happens except that the benefit may last longer.

As the joints improve, there is a corresponding reduction in the number of impulses, travelling from the damaged areas to the muscles, telling the muscles to contract; so, clearly, the degree of spasm is roughly proportional to the level of trouble in the joints. The first treatment is usually given very gently as it can be extremely fatiguing for patients. Most feel very tired for some hours, or even all of the next day, after treatment. This is because it tends to upset the sympathetic nervous system, which is already in disarray, and as it has not yet had time to make any marked improvement, the system may actually malfunction even more.

Where can I get this treatment?

Most physiotherapists and some osteopaths have the necessary equipment and knowledge to give the treatment. It requires only a minor modification of methods that are already in use. A detailed description is given at the end of the book (*see* Appendix 2) so that there can be no confusion as to what the treatment actually involves. A number of physiotherapists have attended seminars on the treatment and so are familiar with the exact techniques.

Appendix 1
EXERCISE PLAN

Regular exercise increases the efficiency of the muscle pump, and keeps the muscles in good working order. A healthy body is a fit body, and chronic back pain can be kept at bay with gentle, daily exercise. Everyone needs and wants different amounts of exercise, so I will leave it to you to develop your own individual routine, incorporating as many forms of exercise as you (and preferably your GP) think proper.

The following is, therefore, the barest minimum of exercise which will help to keep the back – and only the back – in good working order. Anyone can do these exercises, whether or not you suffer from back problems. Even if you are able to move just a fraction of an inch, these exercises will help increase movement and flexiblity, and reduce pain.

- *The neck*

1 Turn the head looking from side to side as far as possible six times each way.

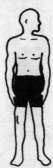

2 Tilt the head from side to side as far as possible six times each way.

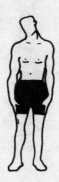

3 Rotate the head keeping the chin to the front six
   times each way.

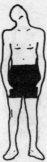

- *The thoracic area*
  1 Rotate the shoulder girdle, with the arms hanging
down, six times in each direction.

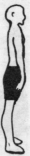

2 Pull the shoulders backwards and forwards as far
   as possible six times.

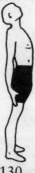

3 Arch the back pushing the shoulders back six times.

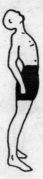

- *The lumbar spine*

1 Rotate the lumbar spine six times with the arms out to the side at about forty-five degrees. At the extreme of each movement give the arms a flick in the same direction to give slight extra movement.

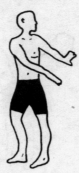

2 Side to side. Lean over as far as possible first to one side and then to the other, six times.

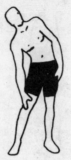

3 Arch the back as far as possible backwards, and then very slightly forward using the lumbar spine and hips as the pivot. Again do this six times each way.

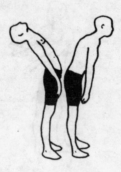

Appendix 2

DESCRIPTION OF TREATMENT FOR THE PHYSIOTHERAPIST

The apparatus and techniques required are as follows:

- **Techniques**. The ability to remobilize and manipulate the back and joints.
- **Apparatus**. Surged faradic machine (preferably as a square-wave pulse) ultrasonic wave generator – any frequency will do but I have found 3M.Hz pulsed the most satisfactory.
- **Massage**. Firm, but not deep, as it must not provoke an hyperaemia.

There is no particular order in which to give the treatment but it may be preferable to use the machines first if the patient is in a great deal of pain as it soothes the tissues and often relaxes some of the muscle spasm. If, however, the patient is not in severe pain, then the electrical treatment tends to relax the patient after the mobilization/manipulation.

Surged Faradism

The surge needs to be set at a cycle of about five seconds. I use pads about twenty-five cm long and five cm wide, and these are placed on either side of the vertebrae to activate the groups of muscles involved. Two or more locations may be needed to cover the whole area of the involved muscle. The intensity should be turned up gradually until it verges on being uncomfortable and then eased back a fraction. It is very important that the treatment is completely pain-free and comfortable; if the strength is excessive it will induce an hyperaemia which will continue after the treatment is over. As a result, instead of the tissue fluids being reduced so that there is a better tissue fluid exchange, the extra circulation will flood the area, defeating the object of the treatment. I have found that three minutes at each location is long enough to serve the required purpose. *Extremely* rarely this may provoke a reaction.

Ultrasonic Waves – Pulsed

This is given for a reasonable period of time at the discretion of the operator. Five minutes over the neck and thoracic area seems a good average. I use from two to three watts per square centimetre (w/sq cm) as this tends to reduce the arteriole circulation and has a maximal effect on the cramp – spasm, inflamed joint, etc.

Mobilization and Manipulation

This is applied to the cervical and thoracic areas of the back. The strength needs careful assessing by test moves and only then should it be employed at the discretion of the operator. A Grade V Maitland manoeuvre (manipulation) or often stronger is often required. I use most of the following manoeuvres:

1. The left thumb is placed with the first joint just below the vertebral spine, comfortably cradling it. The right hand is placed over the left thumb with it fitting comfortably in the hypothenar grove. Press to take up any slack and then push down using the arm and shoulder to give a firm sharp downward and horizontal thrust. All vertebrae should be treated in the area of the muscle spasm at grades V or over.

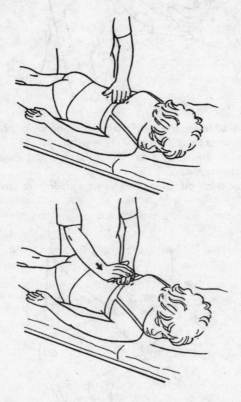

2. With the patient lying on his/her back and the couch head lifted somewhat, cup the chin with one hand and the occiput with the other. Make sure the teeth are closed and the tongue well clear and rotate the head in either direction. One way is almost always more comfortable than the other.

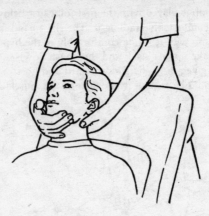

Rotate the head in the *less* comfortable direction using moderate traction at the same time. Take up slack – get the patient as relaxed as possible and breathing right out. Using the arms and shoulders give a thrust about grade V.

Repeat in the other direction, but this time grade V or stronger.

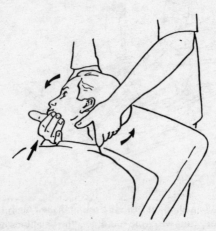

3. Place the patient on his back with the couch flat. The hand nearest you is placed on the opposite shoulder and the other arm brought over it so that the hand is also on the opposite shoulder.

136

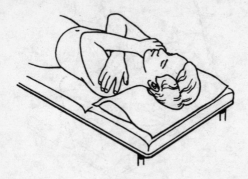

Stand roughly level with the mid chest and lift the far shoulder with your outer arm. Place thumb on the back with a vertebral spine between it and a fist bounded by the first finger.

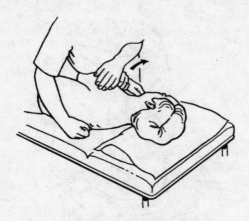

Rest the patient back flat onto the hand and bend over leaning your chest on the folded elbows. Press through the elbows and chest to the vertebrae onto the hand to take up all slack. As the patient breathes right out give a sharp thrust through the elbows and chest.

This needs to be repeated throughout the area of muscle spasm. I vary from grade III in the peripheral areas to grade V and stronger where the back or spines are painful.

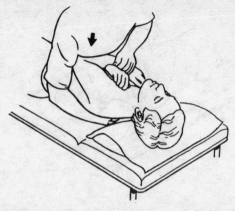

4.   The patient sits on the couch with legs over one side. The buttocks should be well back on the couch. The patient grasps both hands behind the neck or if more comfortable places the hands just on the base of the neck.

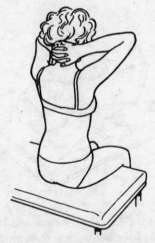

The operator threads his/her arms through the patient's arms and grasps the wrists firmly. The patient leans back on to the operator's chest and becomes as limp as possible. The operator thrusts the shoulders back and his/her chest forward at the same time, loosening the upper thoracic spine.

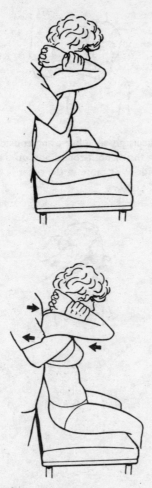

5. The patient sits on a stool with the operator standing behind. Place the left hand on the chin taking special care a) that the teeth are together and the tongue safely out of the way; b) that the inner part of the hand is not or will not press on the trachea which would cause the patient both discomfort and distress. Turn the head both ways – one is usually more comfortable. Start in the other direction.

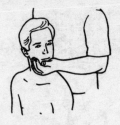

Turn the head as far as possible but using considerable traction at the same time. Give a thrust both round and up – grade III in the first direction and grade V or more in the other.

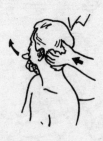

Appendix 3
RESUSCITATION

20,000 people die a year who become unconscious with a heart attack because they are not given the correct first aid
If a person has a heart attack and becomes unconscious it is important to know what to do.

Breathing

The first thing is to assess if they are still breathing: look for chest movement and feel for breath coming out of the mouth, either with the back of the hand or on your cheek. You will need to spend 4 to 5 seconds to be sure of your decision. If at all possible phone for an ambulance as the first priority, because whatever you do subsequently is only buying time before experts arrive with specialized equipment. If you cannot phone for any reason, call for help to send for an ambulance while you attend to the actual first aid.

If the person is breathing, lay him on his back, put the head to one side and lift the chin to ensure a clear airway. (Fig. A.1) *Make sure that you can feel the air coming in and out of the mouth freely.* Movements of the chest are not enough as a guide because these will take place even

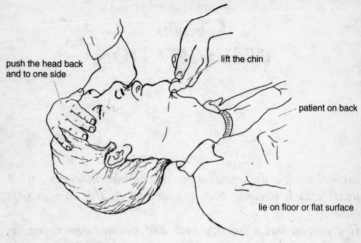

Figure A.1 The Airway

if the airway is completely blocked. Pulling the chin up more firmly will usually restore a free airway and it may need continuous lifting to maintain unobstructed breathing (*see* Fig. A.1)

If the breathing should stop at any time, then artificial respiration should be started.

Heartbeat

As has been discussed, the heart sends a sudden surge of blood into the arteries which expands them suddenly and this can be felt as a 'pulse' in any artery that can be palpated (felt). The wrist, at the base of the thumb, is the place most commonly used by doctors but the easiest place, especially if the operator is at the head end taking care of the airway, is the large carotid artery which runs up to the head (*see* Fig. A.2). It is very readily found

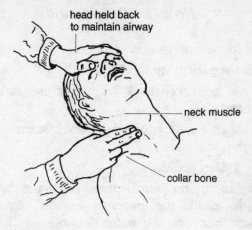

Figure A.2 Carotid pulse

between the voice box and the large neck muscles, just above the collar bone. Practice feeling it on yourself so that you are certain of its exact location.

If the heart is not beating effectively or has stopped there will be no pulse and either condition is regarded as **cardiac arrest** and will normally result in the death of the patient. The casualty may have a good colour at first, but as the blood either drains out of the face he will go pale, or as the oxygen content of the blood becomes used up, the complexion will become blue or grey. The lips have a very thin membrane so the colour is best assessed by looking at them. Prompt, correct measures will save the life of a very large number of these people. If there is cardiac arrest there will also be respiratory failure, so first aid must combine artificial respiration with heart compression to maintain a basic oxygenated circulation of the blood, especially to the brain. This is known as *cardiopulmonary resuscitation* (CPR).

Artificial Respiration

1 Send for an ambulance.

2 Place the patient on the back.

3 Tilt the head well back with your one hand on the forehead.

4 Lift the chin with your other hand but ensure that the mouth is still open.

5 Take a deep breath.

6 Make an airtight joint between yours and the patient's mouth, pinch the patient's nostrils together and breathe out into the patient's lungs steadily over a period of about 2 seconds.

7 Allow the chest to collapse as far as it can.

8 Repeat the process again.

9 If the patient's ribs do not expand as you breathe into their mouth try to improve the airway:
    a) Try pulling the chin up more firmly.
    b) Clear the mouth of any foreign body (dentures etc.).
    c) Try to improve the seal between the two mouths.

10 If the patient resumes spontaneous respiration he should be turned onto his side by bending the arm nearest to a right angle and then pulling his opposite arm across his chest. Then grasp the furthest thigh and pull it over toward you, taking the whole body with it as you roll it onto its side. Keep checking the respiration, pulse and airway. Position the upper knee, thigh and elbow at right angles to prevent the patient from falling right over onto his face (*see* Fig. A.3).

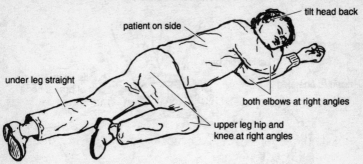

Figure A.3   Recovery position

Cardiopulmonary Resuscitation (CPR)

1 Note the exact time. This can be a very valuable piece of information for the expert team when it arrives.

2 Send for help or get someone else to telephone for an ambulance.

3 Place the patient flat on his back.

4 Give two 'mouth to mouth' exchange breaths.

5 Put the middle finger of one hand in the V where the two sets of ribs meet at the bottom. Put the ball of the other hand's thumb about 5 cms (2 inches) above this, after running it down the breast bone. Then place the first hand on top of the one with the palm over the breast bone and link the fingers (*see* Fig. A.4).

6 Kneel and position yourself directly over the patient's chest with your elbows straight (*see* Fig. A.5).

7 Press very firmly and evenly down, to depress the chest wall by about 5 cms (2 inches) using the 'heel' of the hand – not the fingers. Release the pressure and then repeat the process at as near 80 (almost one and a half to a second) compressions a minute as you can get.

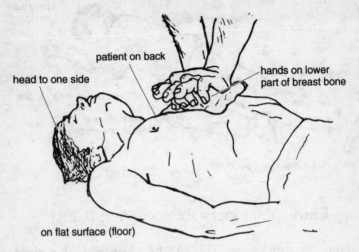

Figure A.4 Cardiopulmonary resuscitation

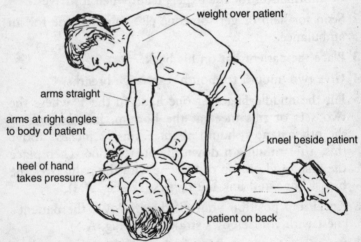

Figure A.5 Cardiopulmonary resuscitation

8 If unaided, give 15 compressions and then two breaths. Keep up this alternation until help arrives or the patient begins to recover.

146

9 If there is someone to assist, one should give the artificial respiration and the other the cardiac massage, both continuously.

GLOSSARY

Acute   Short and sharp.

Adrenalin   A hormone mainly from the Adrenal gland that largely mimics the effect of the sympathetic nerve system.

Alveolus -li   The air cells of the lung.

Angina   Pain.

Angina pectoris   Pain in the chest – heart pain.

Anti-inflammatory   Reduces the inflammatory process.

Arteries   Main blood vessels carrying blood out from the heart.

Arteriole   Small arteries.

Arteriosclerosis   Degenerative condition of the arteries.

Atherosclerosis   Nodules of arteriosclerosis.

Atrio-ventricular node (AV)   Specialized conducting material in the heart.

Atrium auricle   The thin-walled entrance cavities of the heart.

Auricle atrium   The thin-walled entrance cavities of the heart.

Beta-blockers   Substances that block the action of the sympathetic nerve system.

Capillaries   Minute vessels that join arteries to veins, and exchange oxygen and food for carbon dioxide and waste from them to the tissues.

Carbon dioxide   Gas produced by tissue activity which is excreted by the lungs.

Carotid artery   Large artery in the neck, supplying the head.

Catchment Area The area which is drained by, in this case, the lymph vessels.

Central nervous system The brain and associated nerve system.

Cerebral To do with the brain.

Chiropractic Manipulating misaligned bones to restore health.

Cholesterol A variety of alcohol – found in bile, the blood and all cells. It is a constituent of cell membranes, hormones, bile acids, sex hormones and Vitamin D.

Chronic Over a period of time; long-standing.

Clot A semi-solid mass produced by coagulation of the blood.

Collateral circulation Blood vessels running parallel to the one concerned.

Congestive heart failure A slower form of heart failure when fluid collects in the tissue because the heart cannot pump it away fast enough.

Coronary heart disease Disease in the blood vessels that supply the heart.

Coronary Thrombosis A block in an artery that supplies the heart.

Coronary artery Any artery supplying blood to the walls of the heart.

Cortisone Breakdown product of Cortisol, the substance produced by the adrenal gland.

Cramp Painful and involuntary contraction of a muscle.

Diabetes A disease when inadequate supplies of Insulin cause excessive free sugar in the body.

Diastolic The period from the end of the heart contraction to the beginning of the next one. Also therefore the lower blood pressure between contractions of the heart.

Digitalis The dried leaf of the Purple Foxglove (digitalis purpura) used to treat heart failure.

Dilating increasing the internal diameter (or size).

Disc intervertebral The fibrocartilaginous tissue between the

149

bodies of successive vertebrae. It is mainly fibrous on the outside with a soft elastic centre.

E.C.G.   ElectroCardioGram.

Electrocardiogram   A record of the electric impulses generated by the muscle of the heart that gives a great deal of information as to its health and functioning.

Facet joint   The stabilizing joints between successive vertebrae.

Faradism   An interrupted electrical current that is ideal for stimulating the nerves to a muscle. See 'square wave pulse'.

Fibrositis   Pain in muscles and other tissues from inflamed connective tissue.

Ganglion -lia   Collection of nerve cells forming a kind of small 'brain'.

H.S.T.   See HypoSympathetic Tone.

HDL LDL   High Density Lipids and Low Density Lipids are lipoproteins that carry cholesterol to the tissues.

Heart   A muscular organ that maintains the circulation of the blood by its pumping action.

Hormone   Chemical messengers mainly produced by the ductless glands which affect distant tissues.

Hypertension   High blood pressure.

Hypo-Sympathetic tone   An illness newly described that is caused by a lowering of the activity of the sympathetic nerve system.

Hypoglycaemia -mic   Low blood sugar.

Interferential   A form of electrical treatment used by physiotherapists.

Intervertebral disc   The fibro-elastic pad between successive vertebrae.

Ion   An atom, or group of atoms, bearing an electrical charge.

LDL HDL   See HDL LDL.

Lipoprotein   Complexes of lipids with proteins that have many properties of proteins.

Myocardium   Heart muscle.

Occlusion   Blockage.

Oedema   Excessive fluid in the intercellular spaces of the tissues.

Oestrogen   Any substance that mimics the action of the ovarian hormone oestradiol.

Osmosis   The movement of fluid across a membrane to balance an unequal concentration of molecules that themselves cannot pass through.

Osteopathy   Manipulative treatment of joints and soft tissues.

Pacemaker   a) the sinu-atrial node which controls the rate and rhythm of the heart.
b) An electronic gadget inserted to set the pace of the heart after its own control has failed.

Parasympathetic nervous system   A nerve system which has fundamentally the opposite function to the sympathetic nerve system.

Paravertebral   Beside the vertebrae.

Physiotherapy -pist   Treatment by physical means: massage, manipulation, electricity, hot or cold.

Plaque   A flat area, a patch.

Plasma   The fluid part of blood in which the corpuscles are suspended.

Platelets   Flat cells in the blood needed for clotting to take place.

Polymyalgia   Pain affecting a number of muscles.

Prostaglandin   A body chemical messenger. It has many effects, including increasing the inflammatory reaction.

Pulse   A wave of pressure down the arteries caused by the heart beat.

Raynaud's disease   Arterial disease causing extreme reaction to cold, especially in the hands and feet.

Red cells   Cells which give the blood its colour and transport the oxygen and carbon dioxide in the blood.

Serotonin   A chemical messenger found especially in the platelets of the blood, bowel and in the central nerve system.

Sinu-atrial node   (SA) In the wall of the right atrium is the

151

main timekeeper of the heart. Its natural beat is between
60 and 100 a minute.

Sinu-auricular node   Sinu-atrial node.

Spasm   An involuntary protective spasm of the muscle which
is symptomless.

Square wave pulse   A form of faradism that is more
comfortable for the patient.

Stellate ganglion   A sympathetic nerve centre at the base of
the neck that controls a number of functions and organs
including the heart.

Steroid   A group of substances related to cholesterol,
including: sex hormones, cardiac glycosides, bile salts,
corticol, hormones and vit D.

Sympathetic nervous system   An automatic nervous system
that maintains most body parameters and, with adrenaline,
puts it into a state of supreme physical efficiency in a crisis.

Systolic   Related to the period when the heart contracts. It is
therefore the higher of the two blood pressure readings.

Testosterone   A steroid. A male sex hormone.

Thoracic   Chest.

Thrombus   A blood clot formed in, and remaining in, a blood
vessel or the heart.

Tissue fluid   Fluid in the tissues outside and between the cells.

Ultrasonic waves   A very high frequency sound wave, far
beyond the hearing limits of the human ear, that is used
for treatment.

Valve (heart)   There are four valves in the heart: two stop the
blood from going back into the atria when the ventricles
contract, the other two prevent the blood from returning
back into the ventricles when they relax and refill from the
atria.

Veins   Vessels that carry the blood back to the heart.

Ventricle (heart)   The two main pumping chambers of the
heart.

Ventricular fibrillation   Uncoordinated – ineffective

contractions of the ventricles useless to support the
circulation.

Venule   Minute vein.

Vertebra -brae   Individual bones of the spine.

White cells   Disease fighting soldiers of the body; found in the
blood and lymph system, they are the basis of the immune
system.

INDEX

and tiredness, 63
and unconsciousness, 23
figure for, 22
high, 34, 40, 51, 83
in brain, 21
low, 4, 17, 21, 23, 24, 69, 82, 83, 93
maintaining correct, 21, 22, 25, 63
blood sugar, 15
and low sympathetic drive; a *see also* hypoglycaemia
blood vessels, 15, 22, 51
bowel, large, 15, 24, 49, 50
brain, 15
and alcohol, 88–9
and stresss, 44
blood pressure in, 21
development of, 88
stem of, 79
breathing, 14, 25
checking of, 141
bronchus, 49, 50
butter, 40
bypass operation, 59

capillaries, 15, 16, 22, 23, 25, 26, 72
cardiopulmonary resuscitation (CPR), 143, 145–7
cardiovascular system, 7
carotid artery, 23, 24, 50, 142–3
'carotid body', 24
case histories, 20, 21, 39, 43, 54–5, 76–7, 80–1, 82–3, 85–6, 90–1, 95–7, 98–9, 101–2, 106–7, 119–21, 122–3, 124–5
cell combustion, 11
cells
development of in sea 7–8, 9
digestion, 7, 9
feeding, 7, 9
nerve networks between, 9
see also flatworms; roundworms
central nervous system, 48
cerebral arteries, 55

and athero clerosis, 56
and strokes, 56, 97
cervical vertebrae, 70
chest pain, 53, 54, 82, 124
cholesterol, 59–60
and athero clerosis, 59
and diet, 62
and good health, 59
and plasma membranes, 59
and steroids, 59
deposits in arterial walls, 59
in animal fats, 62–3
in egg yolks, 63
levels in blood, 59, 62
chronic food allergy, and coffee consumption, 42
chronic heart disease, 33–4
chronic bronchitis,
and smoking, 44
clots & clotting, 1, 2, 3
and arterial disease, 64, 65
and arterial spasm, 64, 65
and heart attack, 65
and non-return valves, 65
and platelets, 57
of arteries, 44, 47, 57, 65, 96
process of 57, 64, 118
coccyx, 70
coffee consumption
and blood pressure, 41
and chronic food allergy, 42
and coronary thrombosis, 41
and depression, 42
and palpitations, 41–2
and tiredness, 42
cold, as form of treatment, 116–18
'collateral circulation', 66
congestion
and exercise, 91
and ionization, 92
and neck muscles, 102–3
and stellate ganglion, 90, 103
and surged faradism, 114
build-up of, 75, 112

162